the handbook of herbal remedies

Comprehensive A-Z reference guide to over 70 common
ailments from anxiety, digestion, insect bites, to colds, flu,
skin health & wound healing

Heather Dale

medical advice disclaimer

contents

introduction

Welcome to the wonderful world of herbal medicine! As a woman who has experienced the healing power of herbs first-hand, I am passionate about sharing this knowledge with others. Whether you're a seasoned herbalist or just starting to explore the world of natural remedies, this book will provide you with the tools and information you need to promote your health and wellness using the power of herbs.

Herbs are not just plants that grow in our gardens or fields - they are potent allies that have the ability to help our bodies heal and thrive. When we use herbs to treat common illnesses, we are not only treating the symptoms, but we are also addressing the root cause of the problem. This is because herbs work in harmony with our bodies, promoting balance and restoring health.

Herbs contain a wealth of natural compounds that can support our health in a variety of ways. For example, some herbs have anti-inflammatory properties that can help reduce pain and swelling, while others have antimicrobial properties that can help fight infections. Many herbs also contain antioxidants that can protect our cells from damage and help prevent chronic diseases.

One of the great things about herbs is that they can be used to treat a wide range of common illnesses. Whether you're dealing with a cold or flu, digestive issues, headaches, menstrual cramps, or anxiety, there is likely an herb that can help. And because herbs are natural, they are often gentler on our bodies than synthetic drugs, with fewer side effects.

But using herbs for healing is simply not about treating symptoms - it's about taking a holistic approach to our health. When we use herbs to treat common illnesses we are, of course, addressing the physical symptoms, but we are also supporting our mental and emotional wellbeing. For example, herbs such as chamomile and lavender have a calming effect on the nervous system, helping to reduce stress and anxiety. This is why many herbalists believe that herbs can help promote balance and harmony in the body and mind.

I believe that everyone can benefit from incorporating herbs into their lives, whether it's through cooking with fresh herbs, drinking herbal teas, or using herbal remedies to treat common illnesses. Herbs are a powerful tool for promoting health and wellness, and by learning how to use them safely and effectively, we can take control of our own health and live happier, healthier lives.

In this book, I will share with you my knowledge and experience of herbal medicine, providing you with a comprehensive guide to the most common illnesses and the herbs and natural remedies that can be used to treat them. I will explain the properties of different herbs, how they work in the body, and how to prepare and use them safely. Whether you're new to herbal medicine or a seasoned practitioner, I hope that this book will inspire you to explore the wonderful world of herbs and discover the healing power of nature.

The aim of this book is, to simply provide an easy-to-use reference book of herbs that anyone can use - from preppers, to those who simply want to protect and improve general health or who have a specific condition that needs a helping hand or to those of use who are aiming for a more self-sufficient and natural life.

Herbal medicines - from teas to tinctures - have a long-established tradition in almost all cultures worldwide.

Tea allows you to benefit from its medicinal properties and enjoy its soothing effects on the entire body, mind, and soul. It is very easy to make, as long as it takes to boil a kettle, and easy to use (take a sip) and therefore I will focus on herbal teas more than other preparations like tinctures or salves.

This book covers around 100 different conditions with at least 3 or 4 easy-to-use remedies for each one. This means that you can find the one that works best for you - we are all different, and we will all have our preferred herb. My personal favorites are rosemary, sage, thyme, chamomile, garlic, ginger and mint, most of which I grow in the garden (I haven't has success with ginger - yet!)

I have also added information on body systems and the gut microbiome - even a brief understanding of these is invaluable, and I have included an overview in the following pages. Our gut drives almost all health conditions in our body, including our mental health, so its well worth have some knowledge of how it works.

These recommendations are based on a combination of traditional knowledge and scientific evidence, and some sources used in these recommendations include traditional medicine practices and texts, such as Ayurveda, Traditional Chinese Medicine, and other ancient healing systems.

Scientific studies, including clinical trials and observational studies, that have investigated the effectiveness of various herbs and remedies have been the basis of my work, as well as systematic reviews that have analyzed the results of multiple studies to determine the overall evidence for or against the use of specific remedies. It also used guidelines and recommendations from health organizations, such as the World Health Organization and the National Institutes of Health amongst others. And, of course, my own experience. I even use herbs on a regular basis for my dental and oral health.

The purpose of this book is to provide practical information that can be used as a reference at any time. It means that I don't go into detail on the all of the background of the traditions that have delivered us our herbal knowledge and medicine. I have another book that does that!

Like all herbs, you should always check with a medical professional before use, especially if you have a pre-existing condition or are using any medication. Herbs can interact with these and even have the opposite effect to that of which you are aiming for, so remember to respect these plants; they may taste great but they can be powerful! I have included a section on what to watch out for at the end of the book as an example.

For now, dip in and out of this book as you need it, and enjoy this magical world of herbs!

one
your body systems &
microbiome

THE BODY'S systems work together to maintain homeostasis, which is the state of steady internal, physical, and chemical conditions that the body needs to function. This is most often known as balance. Each system plays a specific role in maintaining balance and depends on the other systems to function properly. Here is a brief overview of how some of the body's systems work together:

- The circulatory system transports oxygen, nutrients, and hormones to cells and removes waste products. It works with the respiratory system to exchange oxygen and carbon dioxide.
- The digestive system breaks down food into nutrients that can be absorbed and used by the body. It works with the circulatory system to transport those nutrients to cells.
- The nervous system sends, receives, and processes sensory information. It works with the endocrine system to coordinate the body's responses to internal and external stimuli.

- The musculoskeletal system allows the body to move and provides support and protection for internal organs. It works with the circulatory system to provide oxygen and nutrients to tissues and with the nervous system to coordinate movement.
- The immune system protects the body from infections and other diseases. It works with the circulatory system to transport immune cells and with the digestive system to eliminate pathogens.

This is just a small sample of the ways in which the body's systems work together. Every system in the body plays a vital role in maintaining homeostasis and overall health.

The Circulatory system

The circulatory system, also known as the cardiovascular system, is a body system that is responsible for pumping and transporting blood, nutrients, oxygen, and hormones to, and from, cells. It is made up of the heart, blood vessels, and blood.

The main functions of the circulatory system include:

- Pumping blood: The heart is a muscular organ that pumps blood to the body's tissues and organs.
- Transporting oxygen and nutrients: Blood carries oxygen and nutrients from the lungs and digestive system to the body's cells.
- Removing waste products: Blood carries waste products, such as carbon dioxide and urea, away from the cells to be eliminated from the body.

- Regulating body temperature: Blood helps to regulate the body's temperature by carrying heat away from the body's core to the skin, where it can be dissipated.
- Protecting against infection: The circulatory system plays a role in the body's immune defense by carrying white blood cells and antibodies to areas of infection.

Overall, the circulatory system plays a vital role in maintaining the body's health by transporting oxygen, nutrients, and hormones to cells and removing waste products.

There are many herbs that are traditionally used to support the health and function of the circulatory system. Here are a few herbs that you can use as a tea to support cardiovascular health and improve circulation. These include **Hawthorn** and **Cayenne pepper**. As well as improving circulation, **Ginkgo biloba** supports the cognitive function, **Horse chestnut** can help reduce inflammation and **Dandelion** can support liver health.

The Digestive system

The digestive system is a group of organs that work together to convert food into energy and nutrients that the body needs to function. Our gut, also known as the gastrointestinal tract or digestive system, is a complex system of organs and tissues that work together to break down food, absorb nutrients, and eliminate waste. The microbiome plays an important part here, and this is covered at the end of this chapter.

The gut comprises several parts, including:

1. Mouth: This is where food enters the digestive system. The teeth, tongue, and saliva all work together to break down the food into smaller pieces.

2. Esophagus: A muscular tube that connects the mouth to the stomach. It uses peristalsis, a wave-like muscle contraction, to move the food down to the stomach.
3. Stomach: A muscular sac that mixes and grinds the food with acid and enzymes to break it down further. This breakdown of enzymes is crucial to our health.
4. Small intestine: This long, narrow tube is where most of the nutrients are absorbed into the bloodstream. It is divided into three parts: the duodenum, jejunum, and ileum.
5. Large intestine (colon): This is a wider tube where water is absorbed from the remaining food waste and feces are formed.
6. Rectum: The final part of the large intestine where feces are stored until they are eliminated from the body through the anus.
7. Liver, pancreas, and gallbladder: These are accessory organs that produce and secrete digestive enzymes and other substances into the small intestine to aid in digestion.

Essentially the digestive system maintains the body's health by converting food into energy and nutrients, and eliminating waste products. This is rather a simplistic summary, everything that enters our body (or at least most if it) enters through our mouth, and therefore the effect of our oral health could be a book in itself.

Herbs that support digestive system health (and can be taken as a tea) include **Chamomile**, best known as a calming herb that helps with sleep and relaxation, it has also been used to help with digestive issues. Others include

1. **Ginger**, a warming herb that helps with nausea and inflammation, is also used to help with digestive issues.
2. **Peppermint** can help with digestion and headaches.

3. **Fennel** is used to help with digestion and bloating.
4. **Licorice** helps with digestive issues and can also help soothe a sore throat.

The Endocrine system

The endocrine system is a network of glands that produce and secrete hormones, chemical messengers that help regulate the body's functions. The endocrine system plays a vital role in maintaining homeostasis, which is the state of steady internal, physical, and chemical conditions that the body needs to function.

The functions of the endocrine system include:

- Regulating metabolism: Hormones produced by the endocrine system help regulate the body's metabolism, which is the process of converting food into energy.
- Controlling growth and development: Hormones produced by the endocrine system help control growth and development during childhood and adolescence.
- Regulating mood and behavior: Hormones produced by the endocrine system, such as serotonin and cortisol, can affect mood and behavior.
- Regulating reproduction: Hormones produced by the endocrine system, such as testosterone and estrogen, play a role in regulating the reproductive system.

The endocrine system is especially important for women and women's health and, like all body systems there are many herbs that are used to support its health and function. Here are just a few herbs and teas to try:

1. **Ashwagandha** is used to support the endocrine system and help the body cope with stress.
2. **Maca** is an herb that is traditionally used to support hormonal balance and improve energy levels.
3. **Holy basil** and **Licorice root** can reduce stress and support the endocrine system.
4. **Rhodiola** improves energy levels and supports the endocrine system. Rhodiola is sometimes referred to as "golden root" or "arctic root" due to its golden-yellow color and its ability to thrive in cold, high-altitude environments. Some people also use rhodiola as a natural supplement to improve physical and mental performance, and to reduce stress and fatigue.

The Immune system

The immune system is a complex network of organs, tissues, and cells that work together to defend the body against infection and disease. The main functions include:

- Identifying and eliminating foreign substances: The immune system is able to recognize and eliminate foreign substances, such as bacteria, viruses, and toxins, that can cause illness or infection.
- Protecting against infection: The immune system produces white blood cells and antibodies that help protect the body against infection and disease.
- Remembering past infections: The immune system is able to "remember" past infections and quickly respond to them if they occur again. This is how vaccines work – they expose the body to a small, harmless amount of a virus or bacteria, which allows the immune system to create immunity to that particular disease.

- Maintaining the body's overall health: The immune system helps to maintain the body's overall health by attacking and eliminating foreign substances that can cause illness or infection.

In summary, the immune system protects the body against infection and disease

Here are a some herbal teas that may support your immune system:

1. **Echinacea** helps with the common cold and other respiratory infections and is also used to support the immune system.
2. **Astragalus** is an herb that has been traditionally used to support immune system health.
3. **Ginger**, already mentioned, can also support the immune system.
4. **Turmeric** is a potent antioxidant that has been traditionally used to help with inflammation and pain. It also supports immune system health.
5. **Reishi mushroom** is an herb that has been traditionally used to support immune system health.

The Lymphatic system

The lymphatic system is a part of the immune system and is responsible for the production, maintenance, and circulation of lymph, a clear fluid that helps to protect the body against infection and disease. The lymphatic system is made up of a network of lymph vessels, lymph nodes, and organs, such as the spleen and thymus.

The main functions of the lymphatic system include:

- Filtering lymph fluid: Lymph vessels filter lymph fluid as it flows through the body, removing waste products, bacteria, and other substances.
- Transporting immune cells: Lymph vessels transport immune cells, such as lymphocytes and monocytes, throughout the body to help protect against infection and disease.
- Storing immune cells: Lymph nodes, which are small, bean-shaped structures located throughout the body, store immune cells and produce more immune cells when needed.
- Absorbing excess fluid: The lymphatic system helps to drain excess fluid from tissues and return it to the circulatory system.

As we can see, the lymphatic system plays a vital role in maintaining the body's immune defenses and supporting the health of tissues and organs.

Here are a a selection of herbal tea recipes that can support your lymphatic system health:

1. **Red clover**, this can also help with menopausal symptoms and as a natural expectorant
2. **Echinacea again**, which can be good for the common cold and other respiratory infections.
3. **Calendula**, also used to manage with skin irritation and inflammation.
4. **Cleavers** is traditionally used to support lymphatic system health.
5. **Goldenseal**, also supports the immune system.

The Musculoskeletal system

Once more, here are a few herbal tea recipes that may support musculoskeletal health:

1. Turmeric tea: **Turmeric** is a potent antioxidant that has been traditionally used to help with inflammation and pain. If you are using as a tea then you can also add a pinch of black pepper to help increase the absorption of the turmeric.
2. **Ginger** is a warming herb that has been traditionally used to help with nausea and inflammation.
3. **White willow bark** is traditionally used to help with pain and inflammation.
4. **Devil's claw** is an herb that has also been traditionally used to help with pain and inflammation.
5. **Marjoram** has been traditionally used to help with digestion and to reduce muscle spasms.

It's important to note that these are only a few examples and that other herbs, such as Boswellia and Bromelain, may also support musculoskeletal health.

The Nervous system

There are many herbs that are traditionally used to support the health and function of the nervous system. For example:

1. Chamomile is a soothing herb that is used to reduce anxiety and promote relaxation.
2. Lemon balm is a calming herb that is often used to reduce stress and improve sleep.
3. Passionflower is a herb that is traditionally used to help with anxiety and sleep.

4. Peppermint used to improve digestion and reduce stress.
5. Valerian root is an herb that is traditionally used to promote relaxation and improve sleep.

The Respiratory system

Here are a few herbs that can be used as tea that may support respiratory system health:

1. Echinacea helps with the common cold and other respiratory infections.
2. Thyme and Mullein are used to help with respiratory issues and both act as a natural expectorant.
3. Peppermint helps with digestion and headaches but it has also been used to help with respiratory issues.

If you have a specific problem or are trying to work with a particular organ it is always better to do some research - below are just two examples of the types of herbs that can work with two organs that tend to raise the most questions. In this case always consult with a professional before consuming any herbs by any method.

The Microbiome & Microbiota

Before I end this section, it is difficult to talk about the body systems without mentioning a term you will all know, the gut. Although this is bound up in the digestive system mentioned earlier, the importance of the gut and of gut health cannot be underestimated, and this is where our Microbiome comes in.

Microbiome is the universe of the populations – and all the genetic parts. Microbiota refer the types of microbes or the population including virus' and bacteria. For example the skin has a different microbiota than the gut. These microorganisms include bacteria, viruses, fungi, and other organisms, and they play a crucial role in maintaining our health. The gut microbiota help to break down and digest food, produce essential vitamins and nutrients, and help to protect against harmful pathogens.

In 2004 scientists were surprised to find that we have only about 22,000 functional genes in our bodies, less than an earth worm or even the rice plant – but we have around 3.5m microbial bacterial genes. It means we have more bacterial and viral DNA in our bodies than we have human DNA.

What's more, its estimated that 99% of our metabolic functions – how we breath, how we digest food and even our emotions are coded by this.

It is an entire ecosystem generating energy and vitamins that are vital to us. For example Vitamin B12, Vitamin K come from our microbiome which sits in the lining of our gut.

The intention of this book is to be of practical use, something that you can refer to often and when needed, rather than an in-depth look at the reasons for imbalance in our body and therefore this is a very brief overview of what this all means.

Gut health involves so many health effects, from cancer to constipation to depression and anxiety. Almost everything begins in the microbiome in our gut.

The gut, as we know, is lined with a complex network of cells and tissues that help to protect the body from harmful pathogens and toxins. The lining of the gut, known as the intestinal barrier, is made up of a layer of tightly packed cells that prevent harmful substances from entering the bloodstream. This barrier is also home to immune cells, which help to identify and neutralize potential threats.

Disruptions to the gut microbiota can lead to a range of health problems. For example, an imbalance in the gut microbiota, known as dysbiosis, has been linked to conditions such as inflammatory bowel disease (IBD), irritable bowel syndrome (IBS), and even mental health conditions such as depression and anxiety.

A key factor which can impact the gut microbiota is diet. A diet that is high in processed foods and low in fiber can disrupt the balance of the gut microbiota, while a diet that is rich in plant-based foods and high in fiber can help to promote a healthy gut microbiota.

Antibiotics can also disrupt the balance. Only about 2% of the bacteria that we have in our body is harmful. The other 98% is either needed by our body or has no effect. And antibiotics don't select which bacteria to kill - it kills them all. This can lead to a range of health problems, including increased susceptibility to infections, antibiotic resistance, and the development of chronic diseases.

Recent research has also shown that the gut-brain axis, the complex network of communication between the gut and the brain, plays a crucial role in mental health. The gut produces several neurotransmitters, including serotonin and dopamine, which are involved in regulating mood and emotion. Disruptions to the gut microbiota can lead to imbalances in these neurotransmitters, contributing to the development of mental health conditions such as depression and anxiety.

These microbiota are also important to skin health. The microbiota on and in our skin communicates with the cells in our immune system and can trigger an immune response. It is this that can result in things like eczema, psoriasis and acne.

It means that we need to be aware of what we are eating and what we are putting on our skin. We want, and need, to keep our healthy or 'good' bacteria thriving and many additives including preservers, kill bacteria without selection.

The easiest thing to do is not to overuse antibiotics - it kills all bacteria, don't overuse sanitisers on the skin, and don't be afraid of bacteria.

Some herbs have antimicrobial properties that can help to reduce or eliminate harmful bacteria and viruses, while others have prebiotic properties that can help to feed and support the growth of beneficial microorganisms.

In order to identify which herbs may help for a specific symptom or organs, it is important to consider the properties of the herb and the symptoms or conditions that you are experiencing. For example, if you are experiencing digestive discomfort, you may want to consider herbs with anti-inflammatory or antimicrobial properties, such as **Ginger**, **Turmeric**, or **Oregano**.

If you are experiencing immune dysfunction, you may want to consider herbs that can help to support the immune system, such as **Echinacea, Elderberry**, or **Astragalus**. These can help to stimulate the immune system and protect against harmful pathogens.

If you are suffering from mental health conditions such as anxiety or depression, you may want to consider herbs that can help to support the gut-brain axis, such as **Ashwagandha** or **Holy Basil**. These herbs can reduce inflammation in the gut and support the production of neurotransmitters such as serotonin and dopamine.

In addition to incorporating herbs into your diet, there are several other steps that you can take to support gut health. Eating a diet rich in whole foods, fiber, and fermented foods can help to promote the growth of beneficial microorganisms in the gut. Avoiding processed foods, artificial sweeteners, and other gut irritants can also help to support gut health.

Managing stress, getting adequate sleep, and staying physically active are also important. Chronic stress and lack of sleep can lead to imbalances in the gut, while regular physical activity has been shown to support healthy gut microbiota.

This will all become more apparent as you read through the causes of most of our illnesses - inflammation, a reaction by our immune system, and hormonal imbalance are the cause of most of our problems, and many of them are subsets of the same illness or condition.

In summary, by incorporating herbs into your diet and lifestyle, you can help to restore the balance of the gut microbiota and promote overall health and wellbeing. In some ways, it is that simple.

types of application

In this chapter, we will be taking a look at the many different ways to consume herbal remedies. This includes herbal teas, herbal capsules, tinctures, bud extract, poultices, essential oils, and oil extracts. For each solution, we will discuss what they are, when to use them, and how to create your own. We will cover herbal teas in more detail in the next chapter.

Herbal Teas

One of the most interesting facts about herbal teas is that they are not technically tea. Real tea comes from the tea plant (*Camellia sinensis*) which is responsible for the Chinese, Indian, and Sri Lankan teas that we all know and love.

Herbal teas are perhaps better described as herbal infusions. They are made with hot water and parts of plants or herbs such as leaves, bark, flowers, and roots.

While it may feel like herbal teas are a relatively new addition, they have been used across the world for thousands of years.

A 2021 study published in *Frontiers in Pharmacology* looked at the use of medicinal herbal teas in countries of the Eastern Mediterranean Area (Turkey, Greece, Syria, Lebanon, and Iran) [26].

It found that the teas had been used for hundreds if not thousands of years and are used as a form of preventative medicine. They are used to relax, aid digestion, and as a form of anti-infection.

Herbal teas were used by the Ancient Egyptians, Ancient Greeks and were also used in China and India. Some of the most well-known herbal teas are:

- Peppermint tea
- Chamomile tea
- Rooibos tea
- Echinacea tea
- Lemon Balm tea

But many herbal medicines that are used in different cultures use multiple ingredients rather than just one or two. The study mentioned above notes a Greek herbal remedy that contains 40 ingredients.

As herbal teas are preventative medicine, they can (and should) be drunk regularly, even on a daily basis. It is very easy to research your own mixtures of herbs and roots, which can be done to improve taste, or to provide differing health benefits.

Chamomile tea, for example, is used for relaxation and is famously used to help you fall asleep. However, many people believe that lavender is more effective. Why not combine the two? This mixture of chamomile and lavender can provide an even better sleeping experience.

You can use herbal teas whenever you want. But some of the best times are:

- After a meal, to help with digestion
- During stressful or upsetting times
- Before bed
- As a substitute for a less healthy drink when you feel thirsty
- Socially, people go out for a coffee all the time; why not bond over herbal tea?

You can buy pre-blended herbal teas, or you can make your own. They are surprisingly easy to create. Find a blend that works (check online) and mix the ingredients together (dried) in a bowl. Then store them safely. When you want to brew your tea, take one teaspoon, and add it to a cup of boiled water. If you want a stronger taste, then you can use a larger spoonful of herbs or less water.

In some cases, like Chamomile, if you find the taste too bitter then just removed the leaves and use only the flowers, or add a little bit of honey (I tend to add honey).

The longer you steep the herbal mixture in the water, the more compounds are extracted. You can even leave the herbs in water in the fridge for several hours to increase the strength of the brew.

It is important to note that you don't have to drink teas to get the benefits. This form of water-based extraction can be helpful for creating herbal compresses or as a wash.

Herbal Capsules

Also known as herbal caps or herbal supplements. Herbal capsules are a very common method of ingesting herbal remedies. Herbal capsules are easily compared to pharmaceuticals, but there are several key differences:

- Herbal capsules are not regulated in the same way

- Herbal capsules do not require a prescription
- Herbal capsules can have wildly different ingredients and concentrations

These aren't good or bad things, just something to consider when purchasing.

Herbal capsules can be bought fully-formed, or you can make your own. You can purchase empty capsules online (vegan friendly), and you will need a capsule machine. Then it is all about grinding up the herbs and spices you need and measuring them to fit the recommended dosages.

As you can imagine, making your own herbal capsules is a tricky procedure, and you will want to be certain of the correct dosages and blends. This is not a time for experimenting!

There are many benefits to using capsules to ingest herbs:

- Disguise the taste – While many herbs and plants taste amazing, there are quite a lot that can taste disgusting. Capsules are great for this because they can hide the taste. If you are using a capsule but *want* to taste the herb, too, you can roll the capsule in some of the powder before storage.
- Convenience – If you are buying herbal capsules, then there is almost no effort involved in ingesting them. You don't have to boil a kettle, you don't need to measure out dosages, you just pop a capsule in your mouth and swallow.
- Easy to swallow – Capsules were invented to be easy to swallow. With no taste or aroma, and a smooth surface, the chances of you gagging or struggling to swallow them are low.
- Faster delivery – Compared to tablets, capsules can break down faster, making them perfect for immediate release.

Before taking herbal capsules, you really want to talk to a practitioner. This goes double if you want to make your own. Most herbal capsules, particularly single-ingredient capsules, are perfectly safe. But it is always better to be cautious.

Herbal Tinctures

Herbal tinctures are similar to herbal teas, but they are stronger, and instead of being soaked in hot water, they are soaked in vinegar or (more commonly) alcohol. The alcohol or vinegar will extract the healthy compounds from bark or leaves (or sometimes berries).

This is more effective method at extracting compounds because almost all compounds are soluble in alcohol, compared to only some compounds that are water soluble.

If you are using leaves, then you want them to be dehydrated or dried beforehand. Fill a jar with your dried herb, push it down hard, then fill the jar with enough alcohol (vodka works well) until the herb is fully submerged.

If you are using a potentially toxic herb, you need to measure the herb beforehand so as to avoid toxicity. Although, if you are considering this, it is best to buy a ready-made tincture from a respected herbalist that you can trust. Or just play it very safe and use considerably less than what is deemed toxic.

Once you have created your tincture, you want to store it for at least a month. This will give it all the time it needs to extract the beneficial compounds from the plant. Then you will pour the mixture into a filter and into a jar so that all that is left is the liquid.

Place the liquid into small bottles, and then use a couple of drops on the tongue. The number of drops you use is based on:

- The plant used in the tincture
- Your height and weight
- Your gender
- Your experience with tinctures (you can build a tolerance to some tinctures)

As with capsules, you should really learn how to make tinctures from a well-respected herbalist before making your own. When you *do* make your own, start off with the safest and most benign tinctures, and you can increase the difficulty as your experience grows. Here are some common tinctures that are used:

- Tincture of Echinacea – Used to reduce the symptoms of common colds
- Tincture 0f Turmeric – Used as an anti-inflammatory
- Tincture of Arnica – Used to treat muscular injuries and bruises
- Tincture of Cannabis (usually CBD, so no THC, which causes the psychoactive "high" most people associate with cannabis). – Used to treat stress, anxiety, and inflammation

Herbal tinctures have been used for thousands of years, and they are a staple of herbal medicine. They work very well at treating minor medical complaints such as muscular injury, common colds, and bruising. But they can also be used for more serious issues such as stress, anxiety, and inflammatory illnesses such as arthritis.

Oil Extracts

An oil extract is made in a strikingly similar way to a tincture. You find your plant or herb and place it in a jar. But instead of then filling the jar with alcohol or vinegar, you fill the jar with oil. Virgin olive oil is preferable, but most oils will work fine.

You want to cover the herb or plant in oil but still have a gap between the top of the oil and the jar's lid. Store the oil for six weeks or so, and then filter the oil into a jar so that you separate all the oil from the plant or herb. This can also be done with bark, berries, and roots.

Once you have separated the oil, you can either use it straight away on your skin, or you can turn it into a salve or balm, which is easier to use and to transport/store.

Oil extracts are very gentle, particularly when you compare them to essential oils. This is a great product to experiment with if you are new to herbal medicine, though care should still be taken when choosing which herbs to use.

Here are some examples of great herbs/plants to use for oil extracts:

- Citrus peel
- Lavender
- Rosemary
- Calendula flowers
- Daisies

Salves

A salve is a topical medicine that is used for minor skin infections and abrasions. It is made by mixing wax (beeswax usually) with oil. This oil can be an essential oil (see below), or it can be an oil extract (see previous entry).

Making your own salves is very simple. You need a small amount of wax and quite a lot of oil. Herbalist Bevin Cohen recommends a ratio of 1.25 oz beeswax to 16 oz oil by volume. To make the salve more liquid, you can increase the oil to wax ratio. Conversely, adding more wax (or less oil) will provide a more solid salve or a balm.

Using the oil extracts from before (citrus peel, lavender, etc.) will make excellent salves and balms.

Poultices

Poultices are hard to describe. They consist of a paste made from herbs or plants. The paste is made to be both wet and warm. You place this paste onto a cloth or bandage and then place it over your skin. Poultices are used mainly for minor wound healing, but historically they were used for much larger wounds and injuries.

Poultices can be used for reducing infection, and they can have antibacterial properties (depending on what herbs are used).

The terms poultice and salves are often used interchangeably. This is understandable as they are both used in similar ways (topically to treat minor wounds and infections). But salves are wax-based and are quite weak, whereas poultices are pastes and are stronger.

While poultices are now made from pastes of different herbs and spices, historically, they used to be made from mud or clay. Surprisingly, the clay used in Ancient times may have had powerful medicinal properties.

It would not have been anywhere near as effective as modern medicine but considering this was being used 10,000 years ago, it would have been quite effective for certain injuries.

Common poultice ingredients include:

- Ginger
- Turmeric
- Eucalyptus
- Aloe Vera
- Activated Charcoal

As with salves, poultices require some form of liquid to create a paste. Oil is often used, but milk or water are other common ingredients. Use just enough liquid to create a paste. If you use too much, then it will stop being a paste and won't adhere to your skin quite as well.

Bud Extract

The use of plant buds has its roots in both Ayurveda and Ancient Greek medicine. They are almost identical to the oil extracts we mentioned earlier, but they only focus on the use of plant buds.

A bud can be found in trees and plants. They grow on plant stems and then develop into flowers, shoots, or leaves.

The first recorded bud extract was Acopon, which Galen mentions in his writings in the second century AD. He took buds from the poplar tree and stored them in olive oil for 12 weeks [27]. This balm is still used today to treat sores, bruises, cuts, and even sunburn.

As you can see, bud extracts are prepared in the exact same way as oil extracts for plants and herbs. Fill a jar with bud extracts, cover them in olive oil, wait for 6 weeks or so, and filter into smaller jars. You can then use them to create salves or apply them directly to the skin.

Essential Oils

Essential oils are the most concentrated version of herbal extracts on this list. They are made in different ways to tinctures and oil extracts, but the idea is the same. Extract all of the goodness out of plants, flowers, stems, and leaves into a concentrated form.

Rather than consuming them like you would a tea or tincture, essential oils are often diffused into the air for you to breathe in. This is why they need to be so concentrated.

Essential oils are surprisingly effective for minor medical complaints. They can have antibacterial properties, as well as antiviral and antifungal.

They are best used to aid sleep and reduce pain. Adding them to a bowl of steaming water is a great way to relieve some of the symptoms of a cold.

Essential oils can also be used topically to treat some skin conditions and muscular pain. But you must be sparing with their use. They are also used in many toiletries and can work wonderfully in soaps.

While it is certainly possible to make your own essential oils, this is one aspect of herbal medicine where it makes a lot more sense to just buy the product. There are three ways to make essential oils:

- Steam distillation – Boiling herbs in water until the oils separate and rise to the surface. This method requires quite a bit of expensive equipment and does not produce pure essential oils in any case.
- Expression – Squeezing the oil out of plants using a pressing machine. Again, expensive equipment is required. You get a much purer oil, but it would be ten times easier to just buy the oil you need.
- Expression using solvents – Can't be done at home, only available when making essential oils commercially.

The best option for home use is expression, but you would need a really powerful pressing machine. They tend to cost $200-300, but the best on the market can set you back over $1,000!

While there is obviously a certain satisfaction that can be gained from making your own products, sometimes it makes more sense to buy your products commercially. They tend to be purer, cost a lot less, and are a huge timesaver.

Here are some of the most commonly used essential oils:

- Tea Tree
- Citrus – Lemon, Orange, Grapefruit
- Lavender
- Peppermint
- Eucalyptus
- Camphor
- Basil
- Clove Bud

This chapter is here to help you learn more about the different methods of extracting the good from herbs and plants. Its purpose is not to give you a complete guide to performing each task.

Hopefully, you have a better idea of the different methods of extraction available, and you know how to differentiate between your tinctures and your salves. The rest of this book will be devoted to helping you identify which plants and herbs are effective in the treatment of certain illnesses, diseases, and also some of the minor medical complaints that can affect our lives but first, lets take a more in depth look at the preparation methods of tea.

three
herbs, teas and preparation

WHAT TO CONSIDER Before Creating Herbal Teas

In this chapter we take a more in-depth look at Herbal teas, perhaps better described as herbal infusions or "tisanes." They are made with hot water and parts of plants or herbs such as leaves, bark, flowers, and roots. Additionally, they don't contain caffeine. This makes them different from other teas, such as black, green, and white, all made from the tea plant *Camellia sinensis*.

As fun and healthy as it is to create your own medicinal teas, it's important to consider a few things before you get started. These will help you establish your priorities as well as create a routine that is not only safe but also enjoyable.

Some things you want to think about include the following:

- Are you or the one being treated on any prescribed medications or supplements? This is due to the possibility of negative reactions when combining these treatments.
- What exactly is the ailment that requires treatment?

- Which organs will benefit?
- Are you trying to stimulate any specific emotions?
- Keep the energetics of the condition and person in mind.
  Cold people and conditions require warming herbs, whereas
  warm people and conditions require cooling herbs.

Remember that there is no one way to do something. It is your creation, and as long as done correctly and with caution, you can experiment and make it your own and try not to focus on only treating one symptom. As your herbal knowledge grows, try creating blends that have multiple benefits including treating the desired issue.

Herbs and teas can boost you in many ways because it is a medicine for the body, mind, and spirit. The more intention you bring to the process, the more it will benefit you. However, they are only going to fix certain problems and you or the person being treated may need to make some lifestyle changes like introducing exercise and a healthy diet.

The preparation for almost all herbal teas is remarkably similar.

Preparation

Herbal Tea

To prepare fresh herbs for herbal tea, follow these steps:

- Rinse the herbs thoroughly to remove any dirt or debris.
- Remove any tough stems or wilted leaves.
- Chop or tear the herbs into small pieces to help release their flavors.
- Place the herbs in a cup or teapot.
- Pour boiling water over the herbs.
- Cover the cup or teapot and let the herbs steep for five to 10 minutes, depending on the strength desired.
- Strain the herbs out of the water before drinking.

Steeping time

In the case of fresh herbs two teaspoons should be enough or one teaspoon when using dried herbs.

In general when you see the term 'one part' or 'part' it refers to either the fresh or dried herbs. It's important to remember that the steeping time will vary depending on the density of whatever herb you're using.

For instance, some barks and roots are best when steeped overnight, flowers are good within two hours, leaves can require about four hours, while some seeds can be steeped for about an hour.

Below is a general rule of thumb for the most common herbal teas in terms of how long to steep your herbs. You can soak for longer to get a more robust flavor and sometimes a more potent effect.

- Flowers - 5 to 10 minutes

- Seeds - 10 minutes
- Bark - 10 to 15 minutes

If you prefer a stronger herbal tea, you can use more herbs or steep the herbs for a longer period of time. It's important to note that different herbs may have different preparation methods and recommended dosages.

In almost all cases they are made as follows:

- 1 cup water (8 oz)
- 1-2 teaspoons dried herb (no less than 2 of the fresh herb)
- Honey or lemon (optional)

Instructions:

- Boil the water in a kettle or on the stove.
- Place the herb in a mug.
- Pour the hot water over the herb and let it steep for 5-10 minutes
- Remove the leaves from the mug.
- Optional: Add honey or lemon to taste (or other flavor choice - see below).

There are many ways to make tea taste better, and the best method will depend on your personal preferences. Here are a few common additives:

- Honey is a sweetener that can add a touch of sweetness to herbal tea. It's also a natural cough suppressant, so it can be especially helpful in soothing sore throats.

- Lemon can add a bright, refreshing flavor to herbal tea. It's also rich in vitamin C, which may help to support immune system health.
- Mint can add a cool, invigorating flavor to herbal tea. It's also been traditionally used to help with digestion.
- Ginger is a warming herb that can add a spicy, zesty flavor to your herbal. It can also help with nausea and inflammation.
- Cinnamon is a spice that adds a sweet, warm flavor to herbal tea. It's also used to help with digestion and to regulate blood sugar levels.

The most common flavor mix is honey and lemon but this taste won't work for all teas and tastes.

You can also add your herbs to green tea - There are several herbs that go well with green tea for health benefits. Some options include:

- Mint has a refreshing flavor and can help with digestion.
- Lemon balm has a citrusy flavor and can have calming effects.
- Basil has a sweet, slightly spicy flavor and is thought to have anti-inflammatory properties.
- Ginger has a spicy, warming flavor with anti-inflammatory and immune-boosting effects.
- Fennel has a licorice-like flavor and is often used for its digestive and diuretic properties.

Preparation methods

There are several different preparation methods for herbal tea and the following pages focus on infusions, but here are some of the other popular options:

- Infusion: To prepare an infusion, add one to two teaspoons of dried herbs or two to three teaspoons of fresh herbs to a cup of boiling water. Cover the cup and let the herbs steep for five to 10 minutes, depending on the strength desired. Strain the herbs out of the water before drinking.
- Decoction: To prepare a decoction, add one to two teaspoons of dried herbs or two to three teaspoons of fresh herbs to a cup of water in a small saucepan. Bring the water to a boil, then reduce the heat and simmer for 10 to 15 minutes. Strain the herbs out of the water before drinking.
- Cold brew: To prepare a cold brew, add one to two teaspoons of dried herbs or two to three teaspoons of fresh herbs to a cup of cold water. Cover the cup and let the herbs steep in the refrigerator for several hours or overnight. Strain the herbs out of the water before drinking.
- Tincture: To prepare a tincture, add one to two teaspoons of dried herbs or two to three teaspoons of fresh herbs to a cup of alcohol, such as vodka or brandy. Cover the cup and let the herbs steep in a cool, dark place for several weeks. Strain the herbs out of the alcohol before drinking. Tinctures are usually taken by the drop, rather than by the cup.

It's generally a good rule of thumb to avoid using any aluminum tools and containers with all these preparations.

As herbal teas are preventative medicine, they can (and should) be taken regularly, even daily. It is very easy to research your own mixtures of herbs and roots, to improve taste or to provide different health benefits.

For example, Peppermint tea is used for an upset stomach, headache, irritable bowel syndrome, and even breathing problems.

Chamomile tea is used for relaxation and, famously, to help you fall asleep. But, many people believe that lavender is more effective. It helps with ease upset stomach, gas, diarrhea, insomnia, and anxiety as well as easing stomach upsets, gas, and diarrhea.

Rooibos tea comes from a plant native to South Africa. It is known for its antioxidants and is believed to boost the immune system and help prevent cancer. It may also be good for your heart and help fight diabetes.

Echinacea tea or coneflower is a well-known cold remedy that boosts the immune system and may help with the flu. Don't drink this tea or use Echinacea if you're pregnant, have allergies, or have asthma, and it can also affect how well certain drugs work.

Milk Thistle and dandelion tea are used to help with liver and gall-bladder problems. The main ingredient in milk thistle is silymarin, which may ease the symptoms of hepatitis C.

How Long Will Your Tea Last?

This depends on the type of tea, fermentation method, and whether or not the leaves are undamaged. If a tea leaf is still very much intact and has been well fermented, it will last longer. To get the longest shelf life out of your teas, be sure to store them in airtight containers away from water, heat, and light.

Medical Decoctions

Decoctions are generally the preparation method for denser plant products like stems, bark, roots, and seeds. Many of the desired nutrients are harder to extract than with delicate plant products, so they cannot be drawn out simply using the steeping method. This is why they are best to be simmered in the water to ensure the necessary constituents are effectively extracted - like the iron and copper found in red clover blossoms or the silica found in oat straw. These components cannot be steeped out so they need the decocting method.

How to Decoct Herbs

In a pot or saucepan, add three tablespoons of your desired herb to a quart of cold water. Heat this water at a very low temperature and be sure to cover the pot. Remember that simmering on the heat will likely reduce the amount of water you're left with, so don't be alarmed when you return and find the water is less. Allow simmering to continue between 20 to 45 minutes. You can now strain your water into a jar. Larger batches of decoctions may last as long as a week in the fridge. You can either add a bit of your decoction to juices or infuse with water.

Dosages

The dosage of how frequently you're going to use any of the methods below will depend on the ailment and whether or not your symptoms are improving. It's highly advisable not to use any remedies in place of prescribed medication or in conjunction with prescribed meds as they may interfere with its effectiveness. Nevertheless, if you're treating certain ailments with herbal teas and are unsure of the dosage, let's have a look at some standard recommendations.

How many cups of tea you should drink depends on the condition being treated. Chronic illnesses may necessitate a cup of the herbal tea remedy at least three times a day, whereas severe conditions may call for one cup every 2 hours of awake time.

It's important to use herbal tea remedies for a week before reassessing your condition and ascertaining whether or not you need to continue or seek help.

You may also want to pulse your doses which basically means taking the tea for a certain period of time and then taking a break before continuing again.

How this will look is, if you're using it for 6 days, you would then not use it for one day, and if you're using it for 10 days, you would not use it for 3 days.

Others ways to benefit from herbal tea

Herbal teas contain a wide range of essential nutrients that are also water-soluble, such as enzymes, saponins, carbohydrates, and more.

Though teas are commonly used as a nutritious beverage, many people underestimate their versatility. This herbal remedy is not only for cleansing your insides and preventing internal complications but can also be applied to the skin in a variety of ways.

Below I have included just some examples of the other ways that you can use your herbal infusion.

Steam your face

Facial steams are not only useful to help treat certain skin problems but are also great for simply relieving facial tension, detoxing your skin, and improving circulation which will leave you with an undeniable glow. This kind of treatment is recommended at least once a week (you can do it more if you feel it's necessary). You're going to ensure your hair is tied and won't get in the way and then wash your face as you'd normally do. Then, add about two tablespoons of herbs to a quart of boiling water in a glass bowl and hold your head directly above it. It's important to use a rag or towel to cover your head so that the steam remains inside. You may have to lift the towel every now and then as the steam can be quite intense, but you want to inhale the steam for about 5 to 7 minutes for optimal results. You can pat your face dry with the towel or splash with some cold water after.

- **Lavender** – Soothing and calming. Relieves itching, is astringent, and anti-bacterial.
- **Calendula** – Helpful for those with eczema and psoriasis. It is anti-inflammatory, astringent and anti-microbial.
- **Chamomile** – Helpful for dry, irritated skin. It is anti-inflammatory, anti-bacterial, and has anti-viral properties.
- **White Willow Bark** – calms redness and inflammation and has anti-microbial and anti-fungal properties.
- **Peppermint** – Refreshing, anti-inflammatory and anti-microbial and is helpful for dull, oily, or irritated skin.
- You can use these herbs for most skin conditions.

Baths

There are different kinds of baths, all with their own unique therapeutic benefits. You may not have time for a full body bath all of the time, which is why there are handbaths and footbaths. Each method provides you with the benefits of the tea you're using so don't feel bad when you can only get to a footbath one week and a handbath the following week.

Handbaths

Your hands consist of many nerve endings. Treating these nerve endings can have countless benefits like improved circulation, colds, arthritis, and flu. It can also relieve aches in the hand and symptoms of eczema. Make at least two quarts of tea in a bowl and soak your hands in it (as soon as the temperature is manageable). You can do so for about 5 to 10 minutes.

Sitz baths

This kind of bath can be taken in a regular-sized bath or even in a small basin. Warm sitz baths are good for combating congestion, relieving pains, such as hemorrhoid pain and gynecological issues, and improving circulation to the pelvic area. You'll have to pour your herbal tea mixture into the tub or basin and soak in it for about three minutes. It's best if your entire pelvic section is immersed in the herbal mixture. Cold or cool sitz baths are also good to try as it assists with menstrual cramps, pelvic inflammatory disease, congestion of the spleen or liver and improves functions of the bowel and lower organs, hemorrhoids, and general back issues.

Some people have actually said that alternating between hot and cool sitz baths offers more significant healing and is a great way to remove toxins and draw in nutrients.

You should always start with the hot bath and then move to the cold. So soak in the hot sitz bath for three minutes and in the cool bath for two minutes. This process can be followed three times for the most effective results. It's important to keep warm once you've finished the entire process.

Witch Hazel is believed to soothe hemorrhoids - it is an astringent and anti-inflammatory.

Lavender is great to add to your bath - its calming property is good for anxiety, insomnia and depression - and it smells great!

You can mix these with **Calendula, Yarrow** and **Uva Ursi** - traditionally used to treat any bladder-related infections including Urinary tract infections.

Add you mix to a muslin bag before adding to your bath.

Footbaths

Our feet also contain various nerve endings which is why footbaths can be so helpful to relieve calluses, aching feet, varicose veins, and leg cramps and even remove bad odors. Much like with sitz baths, footbaths don't necessarily have to be hot; you can also benefit from a cold or cool footbath. The ideal foot bath is made with four quarts of herbal tea and placed in a basin where you'll be soaking your feet. If you notice the first symptoms of an approaching cold, you can take a footbath to relieve congestion, headache, and sore throats. Remember to rinse your feet with cold water when you're done, dry them properly, and keep them warm with socks.

Full body baths

This kind of bath has a range of ways you can enjoy absorbing the nutrients from your teas into your skin. You can add the herbs to a sock or muslin, which can be tied to the faucet as you let two quarts of water run through it into the tub, or simply allow it to soak in the water with you. Alternatively, you can make the tea in a container before adding it to your bath water. Your skin isn't the only thing that'll benefit, since you'll be inhaling the nutrient-rich steam too. It's also good for soothing certain skin conditions, and most teas are safe for use in children. Doing so before their bedtime will improve the chances of a good night's sleep.

Examples are:

- Lavender (relaxing - add mint, lemon or rose)
- Chamomile (soothing and relaxing)

Hair washes

This isn't only ideal for a personal pampering session but also helps for treating oily hair, dandruff, dry scalp, and even balding. You're going to use four heaped teaspoons of herbs for every quart of water. Stir it well and allow it to steep for about an hour, ensuring that it's covered. Strain the herbs out and add them to a spray or squeeze bottle for easy application. For extra strength and shine, add a tablespoon of apple cider vinegar to the mixture and begin applying it to your hair. You should focus on applying it to your scalp and eventually saturating your entire head. Allow the mixture to dry on your hair naturally. Herbs for your hair include:

- Rosemary - hair growth, anti-dandruff, itchy scalp
- Nettle - hair growth and scalp health
- Horsetail - scalp health, anti-dandruff, reduces oil in oily hair
- Chamomile - boost shine and hydration
- Lavender - itchy scalp and dandruff

Mouthwashes

The ideal herbs for mouthwash are lemon balm, licorice, plantain, calendula, echinacea, sage, chamomile, or thyme. The preparation is simple because you'll simply be making an infusion and allowing it to cool off before using it to gargle with. The ideal period to continue this process is for about 10 minutes.

Eye drops

Recent years have increased our time in front of cellphones and computers, and this remedy is perfect for treating tired, sore, infected, or inflamed eyes.

The recommended herbs for making eye washes are fenugreek, plantain, basil, chamomile, rosemary, elderflower, thyme, raspberry leaf, fennel, calendula, and red clover blossoms. Since you're making eye drops, you need to make the mixture much weaker than you would for ingestion or for your baths. For every cup of water, add a small teaspoon of herbs, and simmer on extremely low heat for approximately 10 minutes.

For straining, ensure that the strainer is efficient enough to remove even the smallest particles as you do not want any of them getting into your eyes. Now pour the strained mixture into a well-sterilized eyecup and drop it into our eyes. Be sure to blink so that the mixture washes the entire eye and not just one section. You can do this daily to reduce the chances of bacteria getting into your eyes.

Steam inhalations

You'll generally resort to steam inhalations when you need relief from respiratory problems like nasal congestion, bronchitis, coughs, asthma, sinusitis, or to loosen phlegm. Aromatic herbs like oregano, yarrow, thyme, and mint are best suited for this method. You're going to boil one quart of water, and once boiling, remove it from the heat and pour into a glass bowl. Now add four heaped teaspoons of one of the mentioned herbs to the water, lean your head over the bowl, and cover your head with a rag or towel to get as much steam as possible. You can do this for about 7 minutes, but remember to let some cool air in every now and then if the steam is too overwhelming.

Compresses

These can also be used either hot or cold and are useful for a variety of ailments. This basically involves soaking a face cloth or towel in your desired tea mixture, wringing the water out and applying the cloth to the necessary area. Muslin bags are also a good choice. Compresses are ideal for treating skin problems like rashes and infections, improving circulation, relieving pain, reducing inflammation, and more. Cold compresses are best suited for reducing swelling of inflamed areas, and the recommended herb to use is peppermint. Just be sure to keep the problem area warm after treatment, as this prevents feeling too cold. Hot compresses are best suited for arthritic pains, back pains, and sore throats and are commonly used with hot ginger tea. When using a hot compress, you may want to follow up with a brief cool compress.

four
acid reflux

ACID REFLUX, also known as gastroesophageal reflux disease (GERD), is a condition where stomach acid flows back up into the esophagus, causing discomfort and a burning sensation in the chest and throat and can lead to heartburn, regurgitation, and other symptoms. It is estimated that up to 20% of the population experiences acid reflux symptoms at least once a week.

Although there are over-the-counter medicines available, many people turn to herbal teas as a natural remedy. Here, we will explore some of the most effective herbal teas for acid reflux, as well as the reasons why they are effective, and what causes acid reflux in the first place.

When it comes to acid reflux, it's important to consider the underlying cause, of which there are many, that can contribute to the problem. These include diet, lifestyle, and genetics and understanding these triggers can help manage the symptoms. Other than medical conditions such as hiatal hernias or gastroesophage the most common day-to-day triggers are outlined below.

Certain foods can trigger acid reflux by relaxing the lower esophageal sphincter (LES), which allows acid to flow back into the esophagus.

- Chocolate including chocolate milk and cocoa contain a substance called methylxanthine, which can relax the lower esophageal sphincter (LES).
- Alcohol and the caffeine in coffee and tea also relaxes the LES.
- Fatty or dried foods can slow digestions and delay the opening of the LES.
- Citrus fruits like oranges, lemons and limes along with spicy foods, alcohol, tomatoes and tomato-based products all irritate the esophagus triggering reflux symptoms.
- Garlic and onions contain sulfurous compounds that can trigger symptoms
- Carbonated drinks can increase pressure in the stomach and force acid into the esophagus.

In addition to food and drink triggers, there are also certain lifestyle factors that can trigger acid reflux. For example:

- Eating large meals can put pressure on the LES and eating close to bedtime can increase the risk (when you lie down it is easier for acid to flow back into the esophagus).
- Wearing tight clothing or being overweight can put pressure on the LES triggering symptoms while smoking and stress relaxes the LES.

One of the most popular herbs is **Chamomile**. Its calming and soothing properties makes it an ideal choice as it can help to soothe the burning sensations and reduce inflammation in the esophagus. Chamomile also has natural antispasmodic properties, which can help to relax the muscles in the digestive tract and relieve any spasms that may be contributing to acid reflux.

Ginger is well known for its ability to calm the digestive system and reduce symptoms of acid reflux. This is due in part to its natural anti-inflammatory properties, as well as its ability to reduce nausea and promote healthy digestion. Ginger also contains compounds that help to neutralize stomach acid, which can help to prevent acid reflux from occurring in the first place. Some people find that drinking a cup of ginger tea before meals can help to prevent acid reflux, while others may find relief by drinking ginger tea throughout the day as needed.

Peppermint is another herb that is commonly used to help with acid reflux but it is not the best. Peppermint has natural antispasmodic properties that can help to soothe the digestive tract and reduce the frequency of the condition. This is because peppermint has the ability to relax the muscles in the digestive tract, reducing the pressure on the esophageal sphincter and preventing stomach acid from flowing back into the esophagus. However peppermint tea can relax the lower esophageal sphincter too effectively and cause acid to flow back into the esophagus. In this case, drinking chamomile tea or licorice root tea might be a better choice.

Licorice root is believed to help soothe the digestive system and reduce symptoms of acid reflux by promoting healthy digestion and reducing inflammation in the digestive tract.

Like Ginger, Licorice root also contains natural compounds that have been shown to help neutralize stomach acid. You can opt to drink Licorice root tea before meals or throughout the day as needed.

You can also try Marshmallow root or Slippery Elm tea.

While these herbs are generally considered effective, it's important to keep in mind that not all herbs are right for everyone and that hat while these herbal teas can be helpful for digestive problems, they are not a cure-all.

five
addiction

ADDICTION HAS MANY CAUSES, and it can turn up in many different forms. Some people are specifically addicted to one substance (nicotine, for example) yet display no other addictive behaviors. While others may find that they are likely to become addicted to numerous stimuli.

Addiction is partly genetic, partly environmental (if you live next to a casino, you are more likely to develop a gambling addiction than someone who doesn't). It is also circumstantial or can result from trauma (drinking to forget, for example).

Treatment for addiction should involve multiple approaches, and the first person you should talk to is your doctor. Finding the right treatment for your personal requirements is important. For example, a 10-year addiction to heroin is going to have a different treatment to an addiction to nicotine.

Some methods for addiction treatment include:

- Therapy
- Detox
- Group therapy (12 step program)
- CBT
- Medication

Herbal medicine is not going to try and replace the first four treatment methods, but it may work well alongside them. Whether you choose to use pharmaceutical medication or herbal medication is a discussion that you should have with your doctor. But there are certainly herbal options that you can consider.

A 2016 study titled medicinal plants and addiction treatment identified 12 herbs that may aid in addiction treatment. These were:

- Ginseng
- Passion flower
- Caulis Sinomenii (Qing Feng Teng)
- Camellia sinensis (Green tea)
- Nigella Sativa (black cumin)
- Peganum harmala
- Chamomile
- Datura
- Berberis
- Valerian
- Asafetida
- L-Tetrahydropalmatine

Of these 12 herbs, only a few would count as herbal medicine. For example, while chamomile is a common herbal remedy, it was used alongside morphine to treat addiction. There doesn't appear to be any evidence that chamomile alone can cure addiction, but research is limited so far.

Ginseng, **Passion flower**, and **Nigella sativa** appear to be quite effective in treating addiction, while **Valerian root** can help with anxiety which affects withdrawal symptoms and addiction.

Ginseng can be consumed in a tea and may be effective at treating alcohol or opiate addiction. Passion flower can also be made into tea. Valerian root works well as a herbal supplement, while Nigella Sativa works as either a herbal supplement or essential oil.

six
allergies

WHEN A PERSON with an allergy is exposed to an allergen (such as pollen, dust, food, or pet dander), the body's immune system overreacts and releases histamine and other chemicals into the bloodstream. This results in a range of symptoms, including itching, redness, swelling, sneezing, and runny nose.

The immune system's overreaction is caused by the production of antibodies, specifically Immunoglobulin E (IgE), which are designed to protect the body from harmful invaders. When a person is allergic to a specific substance, their body produces an excessive amount of IgE antibodies that trigger the release of histamine and other chemicals in response to exposure to the allergen.

The symptoms experienced during an allergic reaction are the body's way of trying to remove the allergen from the system. For example, itching, redness, and swelling are a result of increased blood flow to the affected area, which is the body's attempt to flush out the allergen. Sneezing and runny nose are a result of increased mucus production, which is the body's attempt to trap and remove the allergen.

Allergies can also cause symptoms similar to a cold. Allergic rhinitis, also known as hay fever, occurs when the immune system overreacts to an allergen, such as pollen, dust, or pet dander. The immune response leads to inflammation in the nose and throat, resulting in symptoms such as a runny nose, sneezing, and a sore throat.

Licorice root can help to alleviate the symptoms of allergies. It contains compounds that reduce inflammation and inhibit the production of histamine, the chemical responsible for the allergic response. Licorice root can be taken in the form of a tea, tincture, or supplement. However, it should not be used by individuals with high blood pressure or those who are taking diuretic medication.

Nettle is a natural antihistamine that reduces inflammation and mucus production in the respiratory system and it can help to alleviate allergy symptoms like itchy eyes and sneezing. Nettle should not be used by individuals taking blood thinners or with a history of kidney stones.

Eyebright is an herb that can also help reduce inflammation in the respiratory system and alleviate allergy symptoms like watery eyes and sneezing. It should be avoided by individuals with glaucoma or other eye conditions.

In summary, the body reacts to allergies as a result of an overactive immune system that produces excessive amounts of IgE antibodies in response to an allergen. The resulting symptoms are the body's attempt to remove the allergen from the system.

There are several herbs that have been traditionally used to help reduce the overproduction of Immunoglobulin E (IgE) and modulate the immune system's response to allergens:

Quercetin: This flavonoid, from a group polyphenols, is found in a variety of fruits, vegetables, and herbs, including onions, apples, berries, and green tea. Polyphenols deserve a book of their own and are getting more and more interest these days as their health benefits are vast. Quercetin, as well being great for a range of issues, has been studied for its potential to reduce inflammation, improve allergies and has been shown to have antioxidant effects and can help reduce IgE levels.

The fruits, vegetables, and other plant-based foods, that are known to have high concentrations of quercetin include:

- Raw onions have been shown to have some of the highest levels of quercetin, particularly red onions.
- Apples, particularly red apples, are a good source of quercetin.
- Berries such as blueberries, strawberries, and cranberries are also high in quercetin.
- Capers are also a good source of quercetin, with a 100g serving providing approximately 100mg of quercetin.
- Kale is also a good source of quercetin, with a 100g serving providing approximately 80mg of quercetin.

Herbs and teas that have high concentrations of quercetin include:

- Ginkgo biloba: Ginkgo biloba leaves contain high levels of quercetin and are commonly used in traditional Chinese medicine.
- Green tea: Green tea leaves contain quercetin and other flavonoids, including epicatechin and catechins.
- Stinging nettle: Nettle leaves are a rich source of quercetin and other flavonoids, including kaempferol.
- Bilberry: Bilberry leaves and fruit contain high levels of quercetin and other flavonoids, including anthocyanins.
- Elderflower: Elderflower is a good source of quercetin and other flavonoids, including anthocyanins.

In some cases, reducing IgE levels may not be recommended, such as in individuals with a weakened immune system or those with certain autoimmune disorders. In these cases, it is important to consult a healthcare professional for guidance

Other herbs to consider for allergies include the following:

Baicalin: Found in the root of the Chinese herb Scutellaria baicalensis, it has been studied for its potential to modulate the immune system and reduce allergies, and it has been shown to have anti-allergic effects by suppressing IgE production.

Curcumin: The active compound found in turmeric, it reduces inflammation and modulates the immune system.

Boswellia: A herb used for thousands of years in Ayurvedic medicine, it can reduce inflammation and improve allergies due to its anti-inflammatory and immune-modulating effects.

Licorice (Glycyrrhiza glabra): This herb is more commonly found in Chinese medicine is used to reduce inflammation and improve allergies.

Types of Allergies

Hay Fever (Allergic Rhinitis)

Herb/s: Nettle (Urtica dioica) or Quercetin

Benefits

Nettle has anti-inflammatory properties that can help alleviate symptoms of hay fever such as runny nose, sneezing, and itching.

Quercetin (s described earlier) can reduce inflammation and improve allergies.

How to use

You can make a tea by steeping dried quercetin-rich herbs such as elder-flower or ginkgo in hot water for several minutes. You can also purchase quercetin supplements and follow the manufacturer's instructions for use.

When not to use

If you are pregnant or breastfeeding, it is best to avoid quercetin as there is limited research on its safety during these times. If you are taking any blood thinners, it is also best to avoid quercetin as it may increase the risk of bleeding.

People who have a known sensitivity to nettle should avoid using it.

Asthma

Herb/s: Baicalin, Mullein, Eucalyptus, Thyme

Benefits

Baicalin is a flavonoid found in the root of the Chinese herb Scutellaria baicalensis.

You can make a tea by steeping dried Scutellaria baicalensis root in hot water for several minutes.

Licorice, Mullein, Ginger, Eucalyptus and Thyme as teas are used to help with respiratory issues and asthma (and to soothe the throat). As well as helping with nausea and inflammation.

How to use

As well as teas, you can also purchase baicalin supplements and follow the manufacturer's instructions for use.

When not to use

If you are taking any medications that affect the liver, it is best to avoid baicalin as it may increase the risk of liver toxicity. If you are pregnant or breastfeeding, it is also best to avoid baicalin as there is limited research on its safety during these times.

Allergic Dermatitis (Skin Allergies)

Herb/s: Curcumin and Calendula

Benefits

Curcumin is the active compound found in turmeric which reduces inflammation and modulate the immune system.

Calendula has anti-inflammatory and antimicrobial properties that can help soothe itching and reduce redness associated with skin allergies.

How to use

You can add turmeric powder to boiling water and steep for several minutes to make a tea or you can also purchase curcumin supplements. As always, follow the manufacturer's instructions for use.

For Calendula - you can make tea using the standard method.

When not to use

If you are taking any blood thinners, it is best to avoid curcumin as it may increase the risk of bleeding. If you are pregnant or breastfeeding, it is also best to avoid curcumin.

People with a known sensitivity to marigold should avoid using calendula.

Food Allergies

Herb/s: Boswellia and Ginger (Zingiber officinale)

Benefits

Boswellia has been used for thousands of years in traditional Ayurvedic medicine and has been studied for its potential to reduce inflammation and improve allergies.

Ginger has anti-inflammatory properties that can help soothe an upset stomach, bloating, and nausea caused by food allergies.

How to use

You can make a tea by steeping dried boswellia in hot water for several minutes. You can also purchase boswellia supplements.

Ginger tea is easy to make but it much better to use fresh ginger if you can. You can use the standard tea method or you can try this one for a food allergy.

Ingredients:

- 2 cups of water
- 2 inches of fresh ginger root, peeled and sliced
- 1 tbsp of honey
- 1 tbsp of lemon juice
- 2 cinnamon sticks

Instructions:

1. Add the sliced ginger, cinnamon sticks s to a medium-sized pot.

2. Pour the water into the pot and bring to a boil.
3. Reduce heat and let simmer for 10-15 minutes.
4. Strain the tea into a cup and add the honey and lemon juice.
5. Stir to combine and enjoy while still warm.

When not to use

If you are taking any medications that affect blood clotting, it is best to avoid boswellia as it may increase the risk of bleeding. If you are pregnant or breastfeeding, it is also best to avoid boswellia.

People with a bleeding disorder or who are taking blood-thinning medications, should avoid using ginger and, because it may also increase bile flow, it should also be avoided by individuals with gallstones.

Allergic Conjunctivitis (Eye Allergies)

Herb: Licorice (Glycyrrhiza glabra)

Benefits

Licorice root is used in traditional Chinese medicine and has been studied for its potential to reduce inflammation and improve allergies as well as being commonly used in herbal medicine to soothe inflammation and irritation of the eyes.

How to use

You can make a tea by steeping dried Licorice root in hot water for several minutes. To use it as a wash, soak a clean cloth in the cooled liquorice tea, wring out the excess liquid, and place the cloth over closed eyes for 10-15 minutes. Repeat as needed.

To make a Licorice eye drop, Mix 1/4 teaspoon of liquorice root powder with 1/2 cup of water. Strain and store the mixture in a clean bottle. To use, simply apply 2-3 drops in each eye as needed.

When not to use

If you have high blood pressure, it is best to avoid Licorice as it may increase blood pressure. If you are taking any medications for heart disease, it is also best to avoid Licorice as it may interact with these medications.

Dust Allergies

Herb/s: Nettle (Urtica dioica), Goldenrod (Solidago virgaurea), Bromelain

Benefits

Nettle and Goldenrod are rich in histamine-lowering compounds, which may help reduce allergy symptoms particularly hay fever, which is often triggered by dust mites.

Bromelain is a proteolytic enzyme found in pineapples that has anti-inflammatory properties. It may help by reducing inflammation in the nasal passages.

How to use

Here are a few ways to use nettle and Goldenrod for dust allergies.

To make a tea then use the standard formula - Boil 1 cup of water and add 1-2 teaspoons of dried leaves. Let steep for 10 minutes, strain, and drink the tea as needed.

You can also take a tincture, which is a liquid extract of the herb. Simply follow the instructions on the label for dosing.

Another option is to take either (but not both together) in capsule form and follow the instructions on the label for dosing.

You can also relieve nasal symptoms by trying a nasal spray. Simply mix a few drops of tincture with saline solution, and spray into each nostril as needed.

Bromelain can be taken as a supplement or as a nasal spray. Please note that while Bromelain has been shown to have some potential benefits for allergy symptoms, it is not a traditional herbal remedy and its use for allergy relief is not well established in the scientific literature.

When not to use

These herbs may not be effective for food allergies or skin allergies and may interact with certain medications.

While Nettle and Bromelain are generally considered safe, it can cause side effects in some people, such as skin irritation, upset stomach, and dizziness. Additionally, people with bleeding disorders, who are taking blood-thinning medications, or who are pregnant or breastfeeding should discuss any use with a healthcare professional before using Nettle.

Goldenrod is also generally considered safe, it can cause side effects in some people, such as upset stomach, skin irritation, and allergic reactions. Additionally, people with kidney disease, who are taking diuretics should consult a healthcare professional before using.

If you who are pregnant or breastfeeding always check with a healthcare professional.

anxiety & depression

ANXIETY IS one of the most commonly diagnosed mental health disorders, affecting 284 million people globally in 2017. Anxiety is often conflated with depression and/or stress, but it really is its own unique disorder, with similarities to both.

While both are mental health disorders, they have distinct differences in terms of their symptoms, causes, and treatment approaches.

Anxiety is characterized by persistent and excessive worry or fear about everyday situations. People with anxiety disorders may experience intense feelings of fear, panic, and unease in response to normal or even minor stressors. There is often an increase in the levels of stress hormones, such as cortisol and adrenaline. These hormones trigger the body's "fight or flight" response and can cause physical symptoms such as a rapid heartbeat, sweating, and trembling.

Anxiety disorders can be triggered by a variety of factors, including genetics, brain chemistry, life experiences, and environmental factors.

Treatment may involve therapy, medications such as selective serotonin reuptake inhibitors (SSRIs) or benzodiazepines, or a combination of both.

Depression, on the other hand, is a mood disorder that is characterized by feelings of sadness, hopelessness, and disinterest in life activities. People with depression may experience physical symptoms, such as fatigue, appetite changes, and sleep disturbances, as well as emotional symptoms, such as feelings of worthlessness and difficulty concentrating. Depression can also be caused by a variety of factors, including genetics, brain chemistry, life experiences, and environmental factors. In depression, there is a decrease in the levels of certain neurotransmitters in the brain, such as serotonin and dopamine. These neurotransmitters are responsible for regulating mood, appetite, and sleep, among other functions.

While anxiety and depression are distinct disorders, they can often co-occur, with people experiencing symptoms of both anxiety and depression at the same time. It's also worth noting that some medications used to treat anxiety can also be effective in treating depression, and vice versa. However, the specific treatment approach for each person will depend on their individual symptoms, preferences, and medical history, and should be determined by a qualified healthcare provider.

Anxiety

Everyone can get anxious from time to time, but an anxiety disorder is more serious. It can affect your lifestyle and can lead to panic attacks, phobias, agoraphobia, and social anxiety.

If you are suffering from an anxiety disorder, then your first port of call should be a doctor, preferably one specializing in mental health. However, that does not mean that herbal medicine cannot be part of your treatment.

Chronic stress, such as work-related stress or financial stress, can lead to anxiety. **Passionflower** contains compounds that can increase levels of GABA, a neurotransmitter that helps regulate mood and reduce feelings of anxiety. Passionflower can also have a calming effect on the nervous system, reducing physical symptoms of anxiety such as increased heart rate and sweating.

Chamomile extract has been shown to be effective for anxiety. A 2017 study found that 1500mg of Chamomile extract taken daily was effective for anxiety disorder. There are two types of Chamomile and it is the German type that is most often used for tea.

Lavender when used as an essential oil, has been shown to be highly effective at reducing anxiety. Anxiety can run in families and like Passionflower, Lavender contains compounds that can increase levels of GABA which has a calming effect on the nervous system. It also has a relaxing effect on the muscles, reducing physical symptoms such as tremors.

Adding some drops of Lavender oil to your pillow or placing some in a bowl of water near your bed can help with anxiety late at night and help to prevent insomnia.

Another herbal remedy you may want to consider is **Ashwagandha**, and it has a long history of use in traditional Indian, or Ayurvedic, medicine. 300mg per day has been shown to reduce stress and anxiety. Ashwagandha is an adaptogen that helps regulate cortisol levels, the stress hormone, and has a calming effect on the nervous system. Additionally, Ashwagandha has been shown to improve memory and cognitive function, making it a useful herb for those who have experienced traumatic events.

Medical conditions, such as heart disease or hypoglycemia, can cause feelings of anxiety and can cause physical symptoms, such as palpitations and tremors. **Ginger** can help regulate blood sugar levels and reduce feelings of nausea and for conditions such as hypoglycemia. Regulating blood sugar levels can help to reduce the physical symptoms that contribute to anxiety.

You might also want to consider **Valerian root** extract; it has been shown to be effective in treating anxiety and stress and is also useful as a sleep aid.

Depression

Depression is characterized by persistent feelings of sadness, hopelessness, and loss of interest in everyday activities. People with depression may also experience physical symptoms, such as fatigue, changes in appetite and sleep patterns, and difficulty concentrating. The causes of depression are complex and can be influenced by genetics, brain chemistry, life experiences, and environmental factors.

While depression and anxiety may seem similar on the surface, they have distinct differences in terms of the underlying causes and the way they affect the body. However, both can benefit from the same herbs and therapies.

There are many causes for depression, and it is beyond the scope of this chapter to list every single one. But many of the causes can be split into three categories:

- Illness and Insomnia – Insomnia can increase your risk of depression. If your thyroid is under-active, you are more likely to get depression.
- •Circumstance – A recent bereavement (for example) could lead to depression, as can loneliness. There are some studies that show loneliness to be one of the leading causes of depression.

- Lifestyle and stress – A highly stressful or boring job has been proven to cause depression. Drinking/taking drugs more often can increase your risk of depression.

Whatever the cause of depression, treatment should always start the same. Talking to a professional or a doctor should be the first step for anyone who feels depressed.

Not only can they help you to identify the cause of the depression, but they can help you map out a route to recovery or at least find a way to reduce the symptoms.

As with anxiety, there are a number of lifestyle changes that you can make to alleviate the symptoms of depression. Here are a few of them:

- Exercise regularly – both aerobic exercise and weight lifting (resistance training) have been shown to boost mood and reduce the symptoms of depression
- Meditation – This can help with insomnia (a common side effect of depression), and it can also help to relax you and reduce anxiety.
- Socialize more - some studies have shown that in as much as 60% of cases, depression is caused by loneliness. Reach out to family and friends or join a group or take up a hobby that involves meeting others
- Sleep more – Increasing the amount of time you sleep each night can have a positive effect on mood. Studies have shown that extended sleep can boost mood and cognition.
- Therapy – Cognitive Behavioural Therapy (CBT) is a well-known method for the treatment of depression; talk to your doctor about this.
- Diet – As with anxiety and insomnia, diet can't specifically treat depression, but it may help to reduce the severity of

symptoms. A diet high in omega-3 fatty acids may help to improve mood, particularly during winter.

If you are currently trying all of the above methods, you may want to consider some of the herbal remedies mentioned below. Talk to your doctor before doing so and discuss ways in which you can incorporate them into your strategy.

In depression, there is a decrease in the levels of certain neurotransmitters in the brain, such as serotonin and dopamine. These neurotransmitters are responsible for regulating mood, appetite, and sleep, among other functions. (In anxiety, there is often an increase in the levels of certain stress hormones, such as cortisol and adrenaline. These hormones trigger the body's "fight or flight" response and can cause physical symptoms such as a rapid heartbeat, sweating, and trembling.)

Today, modern science has provided evidence to support the use of certain herbs for depression and below are just some of the herbal remedies that have been shown to be effective. Most of the following remedies work by increasing the levels of certain neurotransmitters in the brain, including serotonin, dopamine, and norepinephrine.

Serotonin is involved in regulating mood, appetite, and sleep, while dopamine is involved in regulating motivation and pleasure. Norepinephrine, meanwhile helps to regulate the body's stress response.

Studies have shown that 30mg of **Saffron extract** taken daily can be effective in reducing depression in people who are suffering from major depressive disorder. Make sure that the extract comes from both the petals and the stigma.

Turmeric may also be effective in the treatment of depression, but results can take time. Up to 2-3 months! The active ingredient of turmeric is curcumin, and capsules may be an effective method.

Turmeric supplements have lowered depression and anxiety symptoms and depression in multiple trials.

In Ayurveda, there is a herb called **Bacopa monnieri** that is often used to improve memory, but it also appears to have an effect on depression. Studies have found a small (yet significant) reduction in depressive symptoms when taking 300mg daily for 12 weeks.

Historically, **Red Clover extract** has been used for asthma and similar disorders, but there is evidence that it may also be effective for depression and anxiety. Studies in menopausal women found that red clover extract was able to reduce depression by up to 80%. Two doses of 40mg of pure isoflavones are effective, or 5 grams of the whole plant.

St. John's Wort and **Rhodiola** have been shown to be as effective as some prescription antidepressants in treating mild to moderate depression. They work by increasing the levels of neurotransmitters in the brain, including serotonin, dopamine, and norepinephrine.

Ashwagandha is highly effective for anxiety and is best known for that, but it also appears to have some effect on depression. Its ability to reduce stress and anxiety may contribute to its effect on depression. 250mg twice daily (root extract) seems to be the preferred dosage.

There is also evidence that taking **Lemon Balm** supplements can help treat anxiety, depression, and insomnia. Lemon balm is often taken alongside lavender, as the two are thought to have a synergistic relationship.

Alongside herbal medicines, there is a lot of evidence for meditation to be highly effective at reducing anxiety symptoms. Aerobic exercise and resistance training can also have a marked effect. Whether diet has an effect or not is currently being debated, but a good diet can help improve sleep quality which can have an indirect effect on mood.

Perhaps the best way to treat anxiety and depression is through a combination of mental health work (traditional therapy as well as Cognitive Behaviour Therapy), pharmaceuticals (if your doctor recommends them), herbal medicine, exercise, diet, and meditation.

And remember that Native American medicine also believes that your environment and community including your family can have an impact on your mental health. It can make a significant difference to mental health.

arthritis

ARTHRITIS IS a general term used to describe inflammation and pain in the joints. which can be caused by wear and tear, injury, infection, autoimmune disorders, and metabolic disorders.

There are several different types of arthritis, each with their own causes, symptoms, and treatment options. In this chapter, we will explore the causes of osteoarthritis, rheumatoid arthritis, psoriatic arthritis, and gout, and discuss herbal remedies that may be helpful for each type of arthritis.Gout is covered in a later chapter.

Osteoarthritis

Osteoarthritis is the most common form of arthritis, affecting millions of people worldwide. It is caused by the breakdown of cartilage in the joints, which can be due to age, genetics, injury, and wear and tear. The symptoms of osteoarthritis include pain, stiffness, and swelling in the affected joints, as well as reduced mobility and flexibility. The evidence is insufficient to allow conclusions to be reached but some Herbal remedies that may be helpful for osteoarthritis include:

Turmeric contains a compound called curcumin, which has anti-inflammatory and antioxidant properties that may help to reduce joint pain and inflammation. Turmeric can be consumed as a spice in food or taken as a supplement. Acccording to the Arthritis Foundationit is safer to choose curcumin extract because whole turmeric can be contaminated with led. After checking with your doctor, 500 mg capsules twice daily. Also check the standardized amount of curcumin when looking for a supplement, and aim to select brands that use phospholipids (Meriva, BCM-95), antioxidants (CircuWin) or nanoparticles (Theracurmin) for better absorption.

Ginger is another spice that has anti-inflammatory properties and may help to reduce joint pain and stiffness. It can be consumed as a tea, added to food, or taken as a supplement. Studies have confirmed that a daily dose of 500 to 1,000 mg of ginger extract can modestly reduce pain and disability in hip and knee OA.

Willow bark contains a compound called salicin, which is similar to aspirin and has anti-inflammatory and pain-relieving properties. It can be taken as a supplement or brewed into a tea.Some herbal products have been used topically for OA. A 2013 evaluation concluded that Arnica el and Comfrey extract gel might be helpful, and Capsicum extract gel probably is not. The evidence on other products was insufficient to allow conclusions to be reached.

Acupuncture may help relieve osteoarthritis pain and there is some evidence (although small) that suggests that massage therapy may be helpful.

Rheumatoid arthritis

Rheumatoid arthritis is an autoimmune disorder in which the body's immune system attacks the joints, causing inflammation and damage. It can affect people of all ages, but is more common in women than men. The symptoms of rheumatoid arthritis include pain, stiffness, and swelling in the affected joints, as well as fatigue, fever, and weight loss.

While Arthritis and Rheumatoid arthritis can cause joint pain and inflammation, there are some key differences between arthritis and rheumatoid arthritis:

- Arthritis can be caused by a variety of factors, including wear and tear, injury, infection, and autoimmune disorders. Rheumatoid arthritis is specifically caused by an autoimmune response.
- While both types of arthritis can cause joint pain, stiffness, and swelling, rheumatoid arthritis tends to affect multiple joints at once, and can also cause fatigue, fever, and weight loss.
- Arthritis can progress slowly over time, while rheumatoid arthritis can progress more rapidly, causing more severe joint damage and disability.
- Treatment for arthritis depends on the underlying cause, but may include pain relief medications, physical therapy, and lifestyle changes. Treatment for rheumatoid arthritis typically involves medications that suppress the immune system to reduce inflammation and slow the progression of the disease.

Nobody knows exactly what causes this autoimmune disease, but if rheumatoid arthritis is not treated, it can lead to the complete destruction of your joints. There is no cure for rheumatoid arthritis, there rarely are cures for autoimmune diseases, but there are ways to treat the inflammation and soreness. Both pharmaceutical and herbal options are available.

No herbal remedy can cure rheumatoid arthritis, but it can help keep inflammation and pain at bay. They can make up one aspect of treatment alongside:

- Exercise
- Sleep
- Acupuncture (may cause short term relief)
- Western medicine (corticosteroids)
- Mindfulness
- Massage

There are a number of herbal remedies that you can use to lessen the symptoms. Here are six herbs that you can try:

- **Cinnamon** – Studies have shown that cinnamon powder, when consumed in capsules, can help to reduce inflammation. You can also incorporate cinnamon into your cooking if you prefer.
- **Garlic** – Not only can garlic reduce inflammation, but it may also be able to protect the cartilage around your joints. You can use garlic capsules, but it may be just as effective (and a lot more enjoyable) to add fresh garlic to your meals.
- **Willow Bark** – A 2013 study found that willow bark was highly effective in the treatment of rheumatoid arthritis. It contains salicin, which is similar to aspirin, and has anti-inflammatory properties which can help reduce the symptoms of autoimmune disorders like rheumatoid arthritis. It was also found to be effective for several other musculoskeletal disorders. A tincture may work, but tablets of powdered willow bark tend to be most effective. Talk to your doctor before using them.
- **Green Tea** – Another powerful anti-inflammatory, green tea has many uses and is a great drink. You can, of course, take

green tea supplements, but a cup of green tea is always a nice way to enjoy this wonderful herb.

- **Ginger** – The final anti-inflammatory remedy on this list, ginger is a well-known at being effective in reducing inflammation and it can help reduce pain and swelling in the joints caused by the injury. It is best to add ginger into your diet, but you can also consume it in capsule form if you prefer.
- **Cat's Claw** - The Journal of Rheumatology published a study of Cat's Claw for the treatment of RA. Researchers found that in 40 people with RA, the supplement reduced joint swelling and pain by more than 50 percent compared to placebo. You can take as capsules, tablets, and tea. 250 mg to 350 mg capsule daily for immune support. Use products that contain uncaria tomentosa and make sure it is free of tetracyclic oxindole alkaloids (TOAs).

These same herbs can be used for the other forms of arthritis.

As sleep can be such an effective way of reducing the symptoms of rheumatoid arthritis, it may be a good idea to look at herbal remedies to improve your sleep. **Lavender** essential oil is a good start; **Valerian** root supplements can also help.

Acupuncture has been used in Traditional Chinese Medicine for a very long time. Western medicine is still highly skeptical about its abilities, but many people with rheumatoid arthritis swear by it as a form of short-term pain relief.

Psoriatic arthritis

Psoriatic arthritis is a type of arthritis that is associated with psoriasis, a skin condition characterized by red, scaly patches on the skin. (see also the chapter on Skin Conditions).

The exact cause of psoriatic arthritis is not known, but it is believed to be an autoimmune disorder. The symptoms of psoriatic arthritis include joint pain, stiffness, and swelling, as well as skin lesions.

Herbal remedies that may be helpful for psoriatic arthritis include:

Aloe vera is a plant that has anti-inflammatory and analgesic properties and may help to reduce joint pain and inflammation. It can be applied topically as a gel or taken as a supplement.

Turmeric, as mentioned earlier, has anti-inflammatory and antioxidant properties and may be helpful for reducing joint pain and inflammation in psoriatic arthritis.

Gout

Gout is also type of arthritis, which also has its own chapter, that is caused by the buildup of uric acid crystals in the joints, leading to inflammation and pain. It is more common in men than women and is often associated with a diet high in purines, such as red meat, shellfish, and alcohol. The symptoms of gout include sudden, severe pain in the affected joint, as well as swelling and redness. Herbal remedies that may be helpful for gout include:

Cherries contain compounds that may help to reduce inflammation and lower uric acid levels in the body. Drinking cherry juice or eating fresh cherries may be helpful for preventing gout attacks.

Nettle is a plant that has diuretic properties, meaning it can help to flush excess uric acid from the body. It can be brewed into a tea or taken as a supplement.

Ginger, as mentioned earlier, has anti-inflammatory properties and may help to reduce joint pain and inflammation in gout as well.

Prepatellar bursitis (housemaid's knee)

One final condition, and it is listed here because it has many of the same symptoms as Arthritis is Prepatellar bursitis, commonly known as housemaid's knee.

This happens when the bursa sac, a small fluid-filled sac in front of the kneecap which acts as a cushion between the skin and the patella bone, protecting the knee joint during movement, becomes inflamed.

The most common cause of prepatellar bursitis is repetitive kneeling, which can lead to inflammation and swelling of the bursa sac. It means that it is more common among professions such as carpet layers, gardeners, (and, of course housekeepers!) who spend long periods on their knees. Other causes of prepatellar bursitis include direct trauma to the knee, infection, and underlying medical conditions such as rheumatoid arthritis.

While conventional medical treatments for prepatellar bursitis may include rest, ice, compression, and medication. There are a few herbal remedies that can also help and one of the most effective is **Arnica montana**. Arnica has anti-inflammatory and pain-relieving properties and can be applied topically in the form of creams, gels, or oils, or taken orally in the form of tablets or tinctures. It helps reduce swelling and inflammation, as well as alleviate pain and promote healing of the affected area.

Turmeric, due to the anti-inflammatory properties of curcumin, is also effective. Studies have shown that turmeric can help reduce pain and inflammation in the knee joint, and may promote healing. It can be taken orally in the form of supplements or added to food (or even a drink).

Boswellia, also known as Indian frankincense, is another herb that is used to treat joint pain and inflammation. It can help reduce inflammation and pain by inhibiting the production of inflammatory cytokines. Boswellia can be taken as a supplement or added to food.

Ginger is another herb with potent anti-inflammatory properties that can help alleviate the symptoms of prepatellar bursitis.

Other herbs that may be helpful in treating prepatellar bursitis include **Comfrey**, **Devil's Claw**, and **Willow Bark**. Comfrey contains compounds that can help reduce inflammation, while devil's claw has been traditionally used to treat joint pain and inflammation. Willow bark contains salicylates, compounds that are similar to aspirin that can help reduce the pain and inflammation.

As mentioned earlier, there are several conditions that can cause similar symptoms to bursitis. These include Osteoarthritis, Rheumatoid arthritis, Gout, Tendinitis (an inflammation of the tendons that attach muscles to bones. It can cause pain, swelling, and tenderness in the knee, especially when walking or running), and Meniscal tear. This is a tear in the meniscus, the cartilage that cushions the knee joint, which can cause pain, swelling, and reduced mobility in the knee, especially during activities that involve twisting or bending the knee.

blood pressure

MOST PEOPLE HAVE HEARD of high blood pressure (hypertension) and know that it can be dangerous, but few realize that low blood pressure (hypotension) can also be problematic. This chapter will take a look at both high and low blood pressure and identify some herbs that can help.

Before we look at either, we should establish what ideal blood pressure is. Blood pressure is measured in systolic (force that blood is pumped) and diastolic (resistance to blood flow). A good score is somewhere between 90 and 120 systolic and 60 and 80 diastolic.

High Blood Pressure (Hypertension)

The biggest issue with high blood pressure is that it is virtually symptomless. You could live with it for months without knowing. High blood pressure can lead to strokes, heart attacks, heart failure, or even aneurism.

The causes of high blood pressure are varied, but mostly it is the result of living an unhealthy lifestyle:

- Too much salt in the diet
- High body fat
- Lack of exercise
- Not enough fruit and vegetables
- Bad sleep
- Stress
- Smoking, drinking, drugs

The first treatment for high blood pressure should be making lifestyle changes. Eat more fruit and vegetables, exercise more, sleep better, reduce stress. Check out the chapters in this book where we have covered insomnia and stress to find herbal solutions.

There are some herbal remedies that can help to lower blood pressure. **Bacopa monnieri** is a herb that is used often in Ayurveda and herbal medicine. It works by stimulating nitric oxide release, which widens blood vessels.

The wider your blood vessels are, the easier it is for your blood to flow through, and your blood pressure will lower. Take Bacopa monnieri in capsule form.

There is a lot of scientific evidence that **Garlic** supplements can help to lower blood pressure. A 1996 study found that aged Garlic extract could reduce blood pressure by 5.5% in men with hypertension. You can take aged garlic capsules, or you can eat 1-2 cloves of aged garlic per day to get similar results.

Making tea from **Hibiscus Sabdariffa** has been shown to be highly effective at reducing blood pressure. One cup of tea per day with 1 gram of hibiscus is an effective dose. It also works as a mild appetite suppressant, so it could be effective if weight loss is necessary. But discuss this with your doctor first.

Olive leaf extract is another highly effective way to lower blood pressure. This can be taken in capsule form, or it can be drunk as tea. Check the manufacturer's instructions as the strength can differ from product to product.

Low Blood Pressure (Hypotension)

Many people can have slightly low blood pressure without feeling any side effects, and it rarely leads to a more serious condition. However, extreme hypotension can lead to shock, in which case you may need urgent medical attention.

Being dehydrated is a common cause of low blood pressure or having a diet that is deficient in vitamin B-12 or iron. Vegan diets can be deficient in these nutrients, so keep this in mind.

Low blood pressure can be a symptom of more severe illnesses, septicemia, Addison's disease, or heart problems.

While there are herbs such as **Ephedra**, **Ginkgo**, and **Ginseng** that can raise your blood pressure, it is best to talk to your doctor first before experimenting with raising your blood pressure.

bronchitis and laryngitis

As with all herbs and medicine, it is important to get to the route of the illness before treating the symptoms. A cough can be a symptom of many different illnesses, and the treatments for each will differ.

Is the cough due to bronchitis? Is it due to influenza? Is it due to an allergy? Or some form of irritant?

On some level, you should have a pretty good idea of the cause within a few minutes of your cough beginning. If you are 20 years old and run every morning, then the chances of you having emphysema are very low.

You will almost certainly know if you have asthma or a dust allergy or if the five-a-day smoking habit you've had for 30 years has something to do with it.

However, the most common cause for cough is a common cold or influenza (flu). Both come with other symptoms that can help you to tell the difference.

The flu is abrupt; you will start to feel ill immediately. Aches and fever are highly common, as are headaches, chills, fatigue, and weakness. A cough is very common.

Common colds come in stages, with the most common side effects being a sore throat, blocked or runny nose, and sneezing. A cough is also fairly usual.

Acute bronchitis can follow either a cold or a bout of flu and is characterized by a lot of coughing, mucus, and shortness of breath. It usually lasts around 2-3 weeks. Chronic bronchitis lasts for months on end.

You can treat acute bronchitis with herbal medicine; you can also treat common colds and flu with herbal medicine. But it depends on the severity. Anyone with Covid-19, for example, would do well to stick to their doctor's advice due to the severity of this strain. The same goes for any form of flu, and you should probably see a doctor if you have bronchitis too.

One herbal remedy for coughing that has quite a lot of scientific backing is pelargonium sidoides, also known as **African geranium**. It is highly effective at treating the symptoms of acute bronchitis.

It has been shown to cut recovery time from two weeks to just three days for 95% of sufferers. It can also reduce the symptoms of cough in people with acute bronchitis. African geranium appears to be a seriously effective treatment if you have a lingering cough due to acute bronchitis. Use root extract or a tincture mixed with water.

Drinking herbal teas has long been used to treat coughs, and there is a wide variety available. **Thyme** tea can help treat a chesty cough, just add two tablespoons of thyme to boiling water and leave for several minutes to brew.

Marshmallow root tea is another option; it can help with coughs and sore throats. However, too much can lead to an upset stomach, so drink sparingly and stay hydrated.

Ginger is another powerful ingredient to treat colds and coughs, particularly when it is combined with **lemon** and **honey**. Add some chopped ginger, some lemon juice, and a teaspoon of honey to some boiled water and leave to brew for five minutes or so.

A common cough treatment in Native American medicine is Ulmus rubra, also known as **Slippery elm bark**. You can buy lozenges that use slippery elm, or you can make tea from it.

Licorice root is often used to help with bronchitis and laryngitis. To make licorice tea, steep 1-2 teaspoons of dried licorice root in 8 ounces of hot water for 5-10 minutes.

Mullein, and **Eucalyptus** are also used to help with respiratory issues and to soothe the throat. To make tea follow the standard recipe detailed above for Licorice and in the earlier chapters.

burns

Burns can be painful and difficult to deal with, but fortunately, there are many herbs that can help soothe and heal the skin.

First, it's important to understand that there are different types of burns. The three most common types are first-degree burns, second-degree burns, and third-degree burns.

First-degree burns are the least severe and only affect the outer layer of skin. They can be painful and may cause redness and swelling, but usually heal within a few days. A common cause of first-degree burns is sunburn.

Second-degree burns are more serious and can affect both the outer layer of skin and the underlying tissue. They may cause blisters and be more painful than first-degree burns. Second-degree burns can be caused by hot liquids or objects, as well as contact with chemicals or electricity.

Third-degree burns are the most severe and can affect all layers of skin, as well as underlying tissue and organs. These burns are often painless because the nerve endings have been destroyed. Third-degree burns require immediate medical attention and can be caused by flames, chemicals, or electricity.

Now, let's talk about some of the most common problems associated with burns and how herbal remedies can help.

One problem that can occur with burns is inflammation.

Inflammation is the body's natural response to injury, but when it is excessive, it can cause pain, swelling, and redness. One herb that can help reduce inflammation is Calendula. It has anti-inflammatory and antimicrobial properties, which can help reduce swelling and prevent infection. You can use calendula as a tea or make a poultice with fresh or dried flowers. The following herbs are best with minor burns.

Calendula

You can use Calendula in the form of a cream or salve, or as a tea to apply as a compress to the affected area.

The tea made using the standard method - steep 1-2 teaspoons of dried calendula flowers in a cup of boiling water for 10-15 minutes. Strain and drink the tea up to three times per day.

To make a Calendula compress, steep dried calendula flowers in boiling water for 10-15 minutes, strain the liquid, and apply the cooled liquid to a clean cloth or gauze. Apply the compress to the affected area and leave it on for 10-15 minutes, up to three times per day.

Another problem that can occur with burns is infection. Burns can create an open wound, which can be vulnerable to bacterial infections. One herb that can help prevent infection is lavender. Lavender has antibacterial and antifungal properties. Don't apply lavender essential oil directly to the burn, use it in a compress or ointment.

Lavender

- Essential oil: Add 2-3 drops of lavender essential oil with 1 tablespoon of carrier oil (olive oil, to the lavender oil) to create a soothing and healing salve for the affected area.
- Compress: Add a few drops of lavender essential oil to a bowl of cool water. Soak a clean cloth in the water and wring out the excess. Place the cloth on the affected area for 10-15 minutes.

Witch Hazel

Witch hazel is a natural astringent that can help to reduce inflammation and soothe irritated skin. It is great for sunburn and minor burns where it can sooth the skin, reduce the pain and help manage inflammation. Simply add Witch Hazel to a cotton ball or cloth and apply it to the affected area.

Third-degree burns can be very serious and require medical attention. However, herbal remedies can be used in conjunction with medical treatment to help speed up the healing process. One herb that can help with third-degree burns is Aloe Vera. It has anti-inflammatory and pain-relieving properties, which can help reduce swelling and discomfort. You can apply aloe vera gel directly to the burn (if it is not an open wound) or use it in a poultice.

As a rule, if your burn has an open wound, avoid applying herbs directly to the wound as this could introduce bacteria and other harmful substances to the area. Instead, use a sterile dressing or bandage.

Aloe vera

- Gel: Cut a leaf from an aloe vera plant and squeeze out the gel. Apply the gel directly to the burn and leave it on for a few hours. You can also apply the gel and cover the area with a bandage or cloth.

- Poultice: Mash the gel from an aloe vera leaf with a fork or spoon to form a paste. Apply the paste to the affected area and cover it with a bandage or cloth. Leave the poultice on for 15-20 minutes, then remove it and rinse the area with cool water.

While herbal remedies can be beneficial for burns, there are certain situations when you shouldn't apply them directly to skin. As ever, its a good idea to check with a healthcare professional before using herbs for burns.

Below are some examples of when you should avoid applying herbs directly to the skin:

1. If you have a deep or severe burn, you should seek medical attention immediately. Applying herbs directly to the burn could make the burn worse.
2. If you know that you are allergic to a particular herb, do not apply it to your skin. Always do a patch test first.
3. If your burn has an open wound, avoid applying herbs directly to the wound as this could introduce bacteria and other harmful substances to the area. Instead, use a sterile dressing or bandage.
4. If you have sensitive skin, be cautious when applying herbs directly to the skin. Start with a small amount and observe the area for any adverse reactions. If you experience any redness, itching, or irritation, discontinue use.

When applying herbs to the skin, it's important to dilute them first, especially with essential oils. They are highly concentrated and can irritate the skin. Always mix essential oils with a carrier oil, such as coconut or olive oil, before using them on your skin.

cancer

IT WOULD BE impossible to cover Cancer in depth within a single chapter. It is a complex disease that can affect many different parts of the body, and the symptoms can vary depending on the type and stage of the cancer. However, some common symptoms of cancer include unexplained weight loss, fatigue, pain, changes in bowel or bladder habits, and skin changes such as jaundice or unusual moles, and there is evidence that some herbal remedies can help.

Breast Cancer

Breast cancer is one of the most common types of cancer, affecting both men and women. Symptoms of breast cancer can include a lump or thickening in the breast tissue, changes in breast size or shape, nipple discharge, or changes to the skin on the breast.

There are several herbs that may help with breast cancer, including **Turmeric**, **Green tea**, and **Milk Thistle**. Turmeric contains curcumin, which has been shown to inhibit the growth of breast cancer cells and reduce inflammation. Green tea contains antioxidants that help protect cells from damage and may reduce the risk of breast cancer. Milk thistle can help protect the liver, which is important because the liver plays a key role in detoxifying the body and removing cancer-causing toxins.

Lung Cancer

Lung cancer is often caused by smoking or exposure to secondhand smoke, but there are other factors that can increase the risk, such as exposure to certain chemicals and air pollution.

Symptoms of lung cancer can include coughing, chest pain, shortness of breath, and hoarseness. Some herbs that may help with lung cancer include **Licorice** root, **Echinacea**, and **Ginseng**.

Licorice root contains compounds that have been shown to have anti-cancer properties and may also help with respiratory issues. Echinacea is known for its immune-boosting properties, which can help the body fight off cancer cells and reduce the risk of respiratory infections. Ginseng has been shown to have anti-inflammatory and antioxidant properties, which can help protect cells from damage and reduce inflammation in the respiratory system.

Prostate cancer

Prostate cancer is the most common cancer in men, and it is often caused by age and genetics. Symptoms of prostate cancer can include difficulty urinating, frequent urination, blood in the urine or semen, and pain or discomfort in the pelvic area.

Some herbal remedies that may help with prostate cancer include **Saw Palmetto**, **Nettle root**, and **Pygeum**. Saw Palmetto has been shown to help reduce the size of the prostate gland and may also help inhibit the growth of cancer cells. Nettle root contains compounds that can help reduce inflammation and may also have anti-cancer properties. Pygeum is another herb that has been shown to have anti-inflammatory properties and may help reduce the risk of prostate cancer.

Colon Cancer

Colon cancer is often caused by a poor diet that is high in fat and low in fiber. Symptoms of colon cancer can include changes in bowel habits, rectal bleeding, abdominal pain or cramping, and unexplained weight loss.

Herbs that may help with colon cancer include **Ginger**, **Garlic**, and **Aloe Vera**. Ginger has been shown to have anti-inflammatory properties and may also help inhibit the growth of cancer cells in the colon. Garlic contains compounds that have been shown to have anti-cancer properties and may also help boost the immune system. Aloe vera has been shown to have anti-inflammatory properties and may also help protect cells from damage in the colon. Don't consume Aloe Vera unless you are under the guidance of a medical professional who can advise on the appropriate dosage and potential risks.

Skin Cancer

The symptoms of skin cancer can vary depending on the type of cancer and the stage of the disease. Some common signs and symptoms to watch out for include changes in the size, shape, or color of a mole or other skin growth, itching, bleeding, or crusting of a mole or skin growth, a sore that does not heal or keeps returning, and pain or tenderness in a mole or skin growth.

Not all changes to the skin are cancerous, and many moles and skin growths are benign. However, it's important to be aware of any changes to your skin. Skin cancer is most treatable when it is caught early, so be sure to schedule regular skin exams with a dermatologist and practice good sun protection habits to reduce your risk of skin cancer.

There are several herbs that are used to support skin health and may have anti-cancer properties. While some herbs may have potential benefits, more research is needed to determine their effectiveness and safety for treating skin cancer.

All of the following have compounds that have been studied for their anti-cancer effects with some evidence that they may inhibit the growth of skin cancer cells. **Turmeric (curcumin)**, **Green tea** (catechins), **Milk Thistle** (silymarin), and **Aloe Vera** (anthraquinones).

Causes of cancer in the environment

The following list is just and example of some of the things that are thought to cause cancer but this is an ever-developing field and there is now work underway to understand more about the environment impact generally and the impact on our microbiome.

Unsurprisingly tobacco smoke and smoking is a leading cause of lung cancer and is responsible for around 85% of all cases of lung cancer. Smoking can also increase the risk of other types of cancer, including bladder, breast, cervix, kidney, pancreas, stomach, and throat cancer.

Exposure to UV radiation from the sun or tanning beds can increase the risk of skin cancer, including basal cell carcinoma, squamous cell carcinoma, and melanoma.

Arsenic is a naturally occurring mineral that is found in some groundwater and soil. Exposure to high levels of arsenic can increase the risk of skin cancer, as well as other health problems. Arsenic can be found in drinking water, certain foods (such as rice and seafood), and some industrial products.

Polycyclic aromatic hydrocarbons (PAHs) are a group of chemicals that are formed when organic matter is burned. They are found in cigarette smoke, car exhaust, and other sources of air pollution and exposure to PAHs has been linked to an increased risk of cancer including skin cancer.

Formaldehyde is a chemical that is used in many products, including some types of furniture, flooring, and insulation, this too has been linked to an increased risk of several types of cancer.

Heavy alcohol consumption has been linked to an increased risk of several types of cancer, including breast, colon, liver, mouth, and throat cancer.

Exposure to pesticides has been linked to an increased risk of several types of cancer, including leukemia, lymphoma, and brain cancer.

Benzene, a chemical that is used in the production of many products, including plastics, resins, synthetic fibers, rubber, lubricants, dyes, detergents, and pharmaceuticals, has been linked to an increased risk of leukemia.

Asbestos is a group of minerals that was commonly used in insulation, roofing, and other construction materials until it was banned in the 1970s. Exposure to asbestos has been linked to an increased risk of mesothelioma, lung cancer, and other types of cancer.

While exposure to these chemicals can increase the risk of cancer, not everyone who is exposed to these chemicals will develop cancer. Other factors, such as genetics, lifestyle choices, and overall health, can also play a role in determining an individual's risk of developing cancer.

thirteen
carpal tunnel syndrome

CARPAL TUNNEL SYNDROME is a relatively common condition. It occurs when the median nerve, which runs from the forearm to the hand, becomes compressed or squeezed as it passes through the carpal tunnel, a narrow passageway in the wrist that is formed by bones and ligaments.

The symptoms of carpal tunnel syndrome can include tingling, numbness, and pain in the hand and fingers, particularly the thumb, index, and middle fingers. In some cases, the symptoms may extend up the arm. People with carpal tunnel syndrome may also experience weakness in the affected hand, as well as a decreased ability to grip objects.

Carpal tunnel syndrome can be caused by a variety of factors, including repetitive hand movements, wrist injuries, and certain medical conditions like diabetes and rheumatoid arthritis.

Treatment options may include rest and modification of activities that aggravate the condition, wrist splinting, medications to reduce pain and inflammation, and in some cases, surgery to relieve pressure on the median nerve.

Turmeric is a spice that is widely used in traditional Indian and Ayurvedic medicine for its anti-inflammatory and pain-relieving properties. It contains curcumin, which has anti-inflammatory effects that may help reduce pain and swelling in the wrist and hand. A study published in the Journal of Medicinal Food in 2016 found that curcumin may help alleviate pain and inflammation in people with carpal tunnel syndrome. The researchers suggested that curcumin may work by inhibiting the production of inflammatory cytokines, which are proteins that play a role in the inflammatory response.

Ginger is another herb that has anti-inflammatory properties and may help carpal tunnel syndrome. Like turmeric, it contains compounds that may help reduce inflammation and pain in the affected area. A study published in the Journal of Ethnopharmacology in 2015 found that ginger extract may help reduce pain and inflammation in people with osteoarthritis, which is a condition that shares some similarities with carpal tunnel syndrome. The researchers suggested that Ginger also works by inhibiting the production of inflammatory cytokines.

Arnica is an herb that is commonly used topically to relieve pain by reducing inflammation and improving blood flow to the affected area.

Boswellia is generally used to reduce inflammation and pain and it contains compounds that may help reduce inflammation and improve joint mobility. A study published in the International Journal of Pharmaceutical Sciences and Research in 2019 found that Boswellia extract may help reduce pain and improve grip strength in people with carpal tunnel syndrome. The researchers suggested that Boswellia may also work by inhibiting the production of inflammatory cytokines and improving joint mobility.

In summary, while more research is needed to fully understand the mechanisms by which these herbs work, there is some evidence to suggest that they may be beneficial for people with carpal tunnel syndrome.

fourteen
chest congestion

THERE ARE many possible causes of chest congestion, including colds, flu, allergies, asthma, and bronchitis and it can be described as a condition where the respiratory tract becomes clogged with mucus and this is what leads to chest congestion and a host of other uncomfortable symptoms, such as coughing, wheezing, and shortness of breath.

The body produces mucus in response to an infection as a defense mechanism to help trap and remove foreign particles, such as bacteria, viruses, or other pathogens that have entered the respiratory system. The respiratory system itself is lined with mucus membranes that produce mucus, and this thick, sticky substance helps to capture these particles, preventing them from entering the lungs and causing further damage.

The immune response that causes mucus to be produced is primarily the innate immune response. This type of immune response is the body's first line of defense against infections and is responsible for recognizing and responding to pathogens that enter the body. The innate immune system detects foreign particles and triggers an inflammatory response, and it is this that causes the production of mucus in the respiratory system.

In addition to the innate immune response, the adaptive immune response can also play a role in the production of mucus. This type of immune response is specific to the particular pathogen that the body is fighting, and it works to create antibodies that can neutralize the pathogen. As part of this process, the immune system can activate specialized cells that produce mucus to help trap and remove the pathogen.

Allergies, asthma, and bronchitis are all covered in their own chapters and allergies can also lead to chest congestion, as the body produces excess mucus in response to allergens like pollen or pet dander. In more serious cases, chest congestion can be a symptom of asthma or bronchitis, both of which cause inflammation in the respiratory tract, leading to the production of excess mucus.

As a herbalist, one of my go-to categories of herbs when it comes to respiratory issues are demulcents.

So, what exactly are demulcent herbs? Demulcents are a group of herbs that have a soothing and protective effect on the mucous membranes of the body and they are often used to help relieve symptoms of respiratory conditions such as chest infections or phlegm. They contain mucilage, a viscous and sticky substance that has a soothing and protective effect on the mucous membranes.

Mucilage itself is a type of soluble fiber that, when mixed with water, becomes gel-like, providing the protective coating.

When the body produces too much mucus, it can become thick and sticky, making it difficult to expel. This can lead to symptoms such as coughing, throat clearing, and a feeling of heaviness in the chest. Demulcent herbs can help to loosen and thin the mucus, making it easier to expel.

The color of mucus can provide clues about the underlying cause of the condition. While not always definitive, different colors of mucus can be associated with different types of infections or illnesses.

Yellow mucus is typically a sign of a viral or bacterial infection. When the body is fighting off an infection, white blood cells called neutrophils can be released in large numbers. These cells contain a yellow-green pigment, which can cause the mucus to appear yellow. Yellow or green mucus is often a sign that the body is actively fighting the infection, as these colors are produced by the enzymes and white blood cells that are working to eliminate the pathogen.

Yellow mucus can also be a sign of dehydration, as the body's immune system may not be functioning optimally when it is not properly hydrated.

On the other hand, white mucus is typically a sign of a more mild condition. It can be caused by environmental irritants, such as pollution or allergens, or by a common cold or flu. White mucus can also be present in the early stages of an infection, before the immune response has fully kicked in.

It means that, when it comes to the color of mucus, yellow mucus can be an indication of an infection, while white mucus can be a sign of inflammation.

It's worth noting that mucus color alone is not always a reliable indicator of the underlying cause of a condition. Other symptoms, such as fever, cough, and body aches, can also provide important clues about what's going on in the body. For example yellow mucus can be an indication of an infection if it is accompanied by a fever, congestion, coughing, or a sore throat.

Not all cases of yellow mucus are due to an infection. Certain environmental factors, such as smoking or exposure to pollution, can also cause the mucus to become discolored, and some people may naturally produce thicker, yellow or green mucus due to allergies or other respiratory conditions.

For yellow mucus, demulcent herbs that also have antimicrobial properties can be especially helpful. These herbs can help to fight off the underlying infection while also providing soothing and protective effects.

Some examples of demulcent herbs that are good for yellow mucus include:

One of the best examples of a demulcent herb for respiratory issues is **Marshmallow root**. It has antimicrobial properties and is rich in mucilage, making it an effective demulcent for the respiratory system and it has a soothing and cooling effect on the mucous membranes, helping to relieve irritation and inflammation.

Licorice root is also a well-known demulcent herb used in herbal medicine. This herb has a sweet taste and contains glycyrrhizi, a compound that has anti-inflammatory, antimicrobial, and soothing properties. It has been used to help relieve symptoms of respiratory conditions, such as coughs, bronchitis, and asthma and is helpful for reducing mucus production and easing congestion.

Echinacea, while not typically thought of as a demulcent herb, it has powerful immune-boosting properties and can also help to fight off infections that are causing yellow mucus.

Other herbs include **Elecampane** and **Thyme**. Elecampane has antibacterial properties, while thyme is known for its expectorant and antispasmodic properties, which can help to loosen mucus and ease coughing.

To make a Thyme Syrup add near boiling water to 2 tbsp of fresh Thyme (or 2 tsp dried) and steep for 10-15 minutes. After straining add a teaspoon of lemon juice and a quarter of a cup of raw honey. You can take 1 to 2 tbsps every 2-3 hours. The syrup can be kept in the refrigerator for a week.

For white mucus, demulcent herbs that can help to soothe and moisturize the respiratory tract can be especially helpful. These herbs help to ease irritation and inflammation in the airways, while also promoting healthy mucus production and clearance. Some examples of demulcent herbs that are good for white mucus include:

Slippery Elm bark, an excellent demulcent herb for respiratory issues. Like marshmallow root, slippery elm bark is rich in mucilage and has a soothing effect on the mucous membranes and it has anti-inflammatory properties that help to ease irritation in the airways. It has been used for centuries by Native Americans to treat respiratory conditions, such as coughs and bronchitis. Slippery elm bark can be made into a tea or added to cough syrups.

Mullein has a long history of use for respiratory conditions and can help to soothe coughs and ease congestion. It also has anti-inflammatory properties and can help to support healthy immune function.

Plantain is rich in mucilage and can help to soothe and protect the respiratory tract. It has anti-inflammatory properties and can ease irritation and inflammation in the airways.

Licorice root can also be used due to its anti-inflammatory properties.

Reducing mucus production with herbs or other medicines can help to alleviate the symptoms of a chest infection and promote more comfortable breathing. Many herbs have natural properties that can help to thin and loosen mucus, making it easier to clear from the respiratory system.

When it comes to using demulcent herbs for chest congestion, there are a few things to bear in mind.

First, it's important to choose the right herb for your specific situation. For example, licorice root is particularly helpful for reducing inflammation in the respiratory tract.

Once you've chosen your herb, the next step is to decide how to take it. Demulcent herbs can be prepared in a variety of ways, including teas, syrups, and capsules. Drinking a warm tea made with your chosen herb can be particularly soothing, but capsules can be a convenient option if you're on the go.

Herbs can be steeped in hot water to make a tea. This is a common and effective way to take demulcent herbs. To make a tea, steep 1-2 teaspoons of the herb in hot water for 10-15 minutes. Strain the herbs and drink the tea while it is still warm.

Demulcent herbs can be made into a syrup that is easy to take and can be quite soothing. To make a syrup, prepare a strong tea or decoction of the herb, then add honey or another sweetener and cook down to a thick syrup. The syrup can be taken by the spoonful as needed.

For those who don't enjoy the taste of the herbs, capsules are a good option. Demulcent herbs can be purchased in capsule form, or capsules can be made at home by filling empty capsules with the powdered herb.

The recommended dosage can vary based on the herb, the person taking it, and the severity of symptoms. It's always a good idea to start with a lower dose and increase gradually as needed. In general, a common dosage for herbal tea is 1-3 cups per day. For syrups or capsules, the recommended dosage will vary based on the specific herb and the person taking it, so it's best to agree what it best with a qualified herbalist or naturopath for personalized advice.

fifteen
cold & flu

As AN HERBALIST, one of the most common questions I receive during the cold and flu season is about the difference between a cold and the flu. While both are respiratory illnesses and share some symptoms, there are important differences between the two that can affect the severity and duration of the illness, as well as the course of treatment.

Both cold and flu are viral infections. The common cold is caused by several types of viruses, most commonly rhinoviruses, while the flu is caused by the influenza virus. While they are both viral infections, the viruses that cause cold and flu are different, which is why they have distinct symptoms and can affect the body differently.

First, let's start with the common cold. A cold primarily affects the nose and throat, although it can also cause symptoms in the sinuses and lungs. The symptoms of a cold are usually milder than those of the flu and typically develop over the course of a few days. Common symptoms of a cold include a runny or stuffy nose, sore throat, cough, sneezing, and fatigue. It is rare for a cold to cause a fever, and if one does occur, it is usually low-grade.

On the other hand, the flu can affect the entire body, including the respiratory system, muscles, and digestive system. The symptoms of the flu usually develop quickly, within a day or two, and are generally more severe than those of a cold. Common symptoms of the flu include a high fever, cough, sore throat, body aches, fatigue, and sometimes nausea and vomiting.

It's important to note that while the symptoms of a cold and the flu may overlap, the severity of the symptoms is generally much higher with the flu. In addition, the flu can cause serious complications, particularly in young children, elderly adults, and individuals with compromised immune systems.

In terms of treatment, there are several natural remedies that can help to alleviate the symptoms of both colds and the flu. For colds, I often recommend using herbal teas and steam inhalations to help soothe the throat and reduce congestion. **Elderberry** syrup, which has antiviral properties, can also be effective in reducing the duration and severity of cold symptoms.

To make an elderberry syrup you can use the following recipe (or simply make a tea)

Ingredients:

- 1 cup dried elderberries
- 4 cups water
- 1 cup honey
- 2 cinnamon sticks
- 1 inch piece of fresh ginger, peeled and sliced
- 1 teaspoon whole cloves
- 1 lemon, sliced

Instructions:

Combine elderberries, water, cinnamon sticks, ginger, and cloves in a saucepan. Bring to a boil, then reduce heat and simmer for 45 minutes.

Strain mixture through a fine-mesh strainer into a bowl. Press the berries to extract as much liquid as possible.

Return the liquid to the saucepan and add honey and lemon slices. Heat over low heat until honey is dissolved.

Pour into a jar and store in the refrigerator. Take 1-2 tablespoons every few hours as needed.

For the flu, herbs like **Echinacea** and **Ginger** can help to boost the immune system and reduce inflammation. Elderberry syrup can also be effective for the flu, as it has been shown to reduce the severity and duration of symptoms in some studies.

In addition to natural remedies, there are also several preventative measures that can help to reduce your risk of contracting a cold or the flu. These include washing your hands frequently, avoiding close contact with individuals who are sick, and staying home when you are ill to avoid spreading the virus to others.

If you have a high fever, severe cough, or difficulty breathing, it's important to seek medical attention immediately.

sixteen
constipation

CONSTIPATION IS where your intestinal motility (how fast food passes through the intestines) is slowed down for long enough to cause bloating, pain, and difficulty with defecation. Unlike diarrhea, constipation is rarely due to food poisoning, and it is a lot safer to treat with herbal remedies.

Herbal teas are often used to treat constipation and have been used for centuries. Interestingly, constipation is one of the few conditions that can be improved with caffeine, with both **black tea** and **coffee** helping to increase intestinal motility.

The most well-known herbal tea for constipation is **Senna Leaf** tea. The senna leaf has one job and one job only, clearing your bowels at a rapid rate. Senna leaf contains sennosides, which are natural laxatives.

When using Senna, you want to use as little as possible. This is definitely *not* a tea that you want to over consume. Use powdered extract and try the minimum dose of 1 gram. If, after a couple of hours, you are still constipated, you can up the dose slightly and try again.

If you frequently have low intestinal motility, then taking a small dose of senna leaf extract before bed is a good way to regulate your system. It may be a good idea to talk to your doctor before doing this, though.

Avoid Senna if you have kidney or heart problems and if you are trying to get pregnant, already pregnant or breastfeeding. Check and with a doctor before using.

As seems to be the case for most conditions, **Ginger** and **Peppermint** tea appear to be slightly effective in treating constipation. Though they are milder in their effects than senna leaf tea.

Perhaps if you feel slightly bloated and have a mild case of constipation, then they would be a better choice than Senna, which can sometimes work like a sledgehammer to a nail!

Althea officinalis, also known as **Marshmallow root**, is a herb used in European, Asian, and African herbal medicine for a variety of medical complaints and it can aid digestion and will work as a decent laxative.

However, it does have diuretic properties, meaning that you should increase your fluid intake if you decide to use it. Marshmallow root works well as a tea and is best taken before bed.

Constipation has numerous causes, but the biggest ones are not eating enough fiber in your diet, not drinking enough water, and being inactive. Adding a daily walk to your day could make a huge difference to intestinal motility.

Reducing stress can also help. If you suffer from anxiety and depression, finding ways to treat them can also help improve your digestive health.

seventeen
coughs

WE HAVE COVERED coughing as the results of Bronchitis and Laryngitis in an earlier chapter but sometimes we 'just have a cough' and this can be either with mucus or as a dry cough (along with a dry throat).

Mucus production (discussed in Chest Conjestion), and a dry cough are two different aspects of the respiratory system that can be related to each other but have different underlying causes.

Mucus production is a natural response of the body to an irritant, such as an infection, allergen, or irritant in the air. When the body detects an irritant, it responds by producing more mucus, which helps to trap and remove the irritant from the respiratory system. Excess mucus production can cause symptoms such as coughing, throat clearing, and a runny nose, as the body tries to expel the mucus.

A dry cough is a cough that does not produce any phlegm or mucus. It is often caused by irritation in the respiratory system, such as from allergens or irritants in the air, but it can also be due to viral infections, asthma, or other underlying respiratory conditions.

A dry throat and a dry cough are related but not the same thing and a dry cough can be aggravated by a dry throat.

A dry throat refers to a sensation of discomfort or irritation in the throat due to a lack of moisture (and as noted above, a dry cough refers to a cough that does not produce any phlegm or mucus). To address a dry throat, it is important to hydrate the body by drinking plenty of fluids, avoiding dry air, and using a humidifier if necessary.

In some cases, soothing herbs such as **Slippery Elm** or **Marshmallow root** can be used to help lubricate and soothe the throat tissues

For a dry cough, it is important to identify and address the underlying cause, such as allergies or viral infections. As with a dry throat, drinking plenty of fluids and using a humidifier can help to alleviate coughing while herbs such as **Marshmallow root** or **Licorice root** can soothe and protect the respiratory system.

While mucus production and dry coughs are both responses of the respiratory system, they are caused by different mechanisms. Mucus production is a natural defence mechanism of the body to remove irritants from the respiratory system, while a dry cough is a reflexive response to irritation in the respiratory system.

Treatment for excessive mucus production may include the herbs **Mullein** and **Thyme** which help expel the mucus.

eighteen
dementia & alzheimer's

DEMENTIA IS a group of conditions that involve a loss of memory and cognition. One of these conditions is Alzheimer's disease. It is by far the most common form, which is why the two terms are often used interchangeably. But you can have other forms of dementia.

According to research in the National Centre for Biotechnology Information one of the important hallmarks of the aging process is oxidative damage and the neuronal dysfunction observed in disorders associated with aging, such as Alzheimer's disease. Crudely, it is thought to be from oxidative stress and that free radicals are responsible for this oxidative stress. When anti-oxidants are not able to counter the damage that free radicals can do to cells, then we see the effects of aging and related diseases. This is where plant extracts with anti-oxidant and other ingredients might be a great help.

Alzheimer's is a complicated disease and it can't be cured, but you can slow it down. Herbal remedies for dementia are still quite rare, and it should be noted that many cultures that rely on herbal medicine have higher rates of Alzheimer's than cultures that rely on modern medicine.

However, there are other studies being carried out into the use of certain herbs for the treatment of dementia and Alzheimer's. These include:

- **Panax ginseng**
- **Serrate clubmoss** (from which Huperzine A is extracted)
- **Salvia officinalis**
- **Ginkgo biloba**

All four of these herbs are currently being looked at as preventatives as well as possible treatments.

Other research indicates that several targets relevant to the treatment of Alzheimer's disease could be found in **Lavender** (and **Rosemary)** because of the anticholinergic, neuroprotective, and antioxidant activities that lavender displays.

Saffron has also been found to be more effective than placebo, and as effective as donepezil, in clinical trials on anti-Alzheimer effect.

It is important to note that the cause of Alzheimer's disease has not been found, so preventative treatments are hard to come by.

Exercise and diet appear to reduce your risk slightly, and perhaps the four herbs mentioned in this chapter can also offer some protection. Reducing alcohol intake and avoiding smoking also appear to make a difference.

There are other herbs that can improve cognition, and herbs such as **Sage**, **Ginger** and the **Turmeric** may also be effective and there is growing evidence that curcumin (the active pigment found in turmeric) may help to protect against Alzheimer's disease. It works to reduce inflammation as well as the build-up of protein plaques in the brain that are characteristic of Alzheimer's disease.

While most of the current research is being carried out in a lab or on animals, the results are encouraging, and this wonderful spice will continue to be investigated as a powerful tool in improving our health. And it's a great excuse to make a curry!

nineteen
earache and wax

AS WITH TOOTHACHE, there can be a number of causes for earache. In fact, if you are suffering from a dental abscess, you could have toothache and earache simultaneously. How unlucky would that be?

Other causes for earaches can include earwax build-up, a perforated eardrum, a sore throat, tonsillitis, the flu, a cold, or an ear infection.

By far, the most common complaint is caused by wax. If you have a blocked ear due to ear wax then you will have something called 'swimmers ear' which, as the name suggests, feels and sounds like you have water blocking your ear.

This can be caused by using ear plugs, in-ear head phones, hearing aids, hair in the ears, using Q-tips or cotton buds to clean the ears or eczema/psoriasis.

Using in-ear headphones, ear plugs, or hearing aids can disrupt the natural cleaning process of the ear and 'pack' the wax together - and using buds to clean your ears does the same thing - you inadvertently push the wax down into itself.

Excess hair also disrupts the natural cleaning process.

Removing the blockage is very easy. **Almond Oil** (recommended by the NHS in the UK) and medical-grade **Olive Oil** are both effective. Simply put a few drops into your ear daily and this will loosen the wax although it might take a day or two.

If you need to have the wax removed through suction, then use either oil before your doctors visit as it will help to soften the wax, making the removal easier.

If you want to add an antibacterial element, you can mix in some **Tea Tree oil** with your olive oil before adding drops into your ear. This is usually effective for ear infections, but it is advisable to check with your doctor first if you believe that you have an ear infection.

Another option is **Garlic oil**, which offers the same benefits as regular olive oil but also provides antimicrobial benefits that can prevent bacterial or viral infections.

Whichever oil you use, the guidance is the same. Apply a couple of drops to the ear and then lie on your side, allowing the oil to travel down your ear canal. Stay like this for a few minutes and then get up.

After doing this for a couple of weeks, your earwax build-up should have vanished. If you are suffering from other forms of earache that are not earwax-related, then perform the same technique, but you can expect quick results.

If your earache persists for more than a couple of days, then it could well be an ear infection, flu, or cold. Or it could be a perforated eardrum (though this would be obvious straight away). Book an appointment with your doctor.

twenty
diabetes

DIABETES IS a medical condition that occurs when the body is unable to produce or properly use insulin. Insulin is a hormone that regulates the amount of sugar (glucose) in your blood. When you have diabetes, your blood sugar levels are too high, which can lead to a variety of health problems.

There are two main types of diabetes: type 1 and type 2. Type 1 diabetes is an autoimmune disease where the body attacks and destroys the cells in the pancreas that produce insulin. Type 2 diabetes is a metabolic disorder where the body becomes resistant to insulin or doesn't produce enough insulin to keep blood sugar levels under control.

Type 1 diabetes usually develops in childhood or adolescence, while type 2 diabetes is more commonly seen in adults, although it can also occur in children. Other types of diabetes include gestational diabetes, which can occur during pregnancy, and prediabetes, which is a condition where blood sugar levels are higher than normal but not high enough to be diagnosed as diabetes.

The symptoms of diabetes can vary depending on the type and severity of the condition. Some common symptoms include:

- Increased thirst and urination
- Extreme hunger
- Fatigue
- Blurred vision
- Slow healing wounds
- Tingling or numbness in the hands or feet

If left untreated, diabetes can lead to serious health complications, including nerve damage, kidney damage, heart disease, and stroke.

While there is no cure for diabetes, there are ways to manage the condition and prevent or delay complications. Maintaining a healthy diet, getting regular exercise, and managing stress are all important factors in managing diabetes. Additionally, there are some herbal remedies that have been shown to help manage blood sugar levels.

One such remedy is **Cinnamon**. Studies have shown that Cinnamon can help lower blood sugar levels and improve insulin sensitivity. One study found that taking Cinnamon supplements for 90 days resulted in lower fasting blood sugar levels in people with type 2 diabetes.

Another herb that has been shown to help manage diabetes is **Fenugreek.** Fenugreek is a plant that is commonly used in Indian and Middle Eastern cooking. Studies have shown that fenugreek can help lower blood sugar levels and improve insulin sensitivity. One study found that taking Fenugreek supplements for six months resulted in lower fasting blood sugar levels and improved glucose tolerance in people with type 2 diabetes.

Gymnema is another herb that has been traditionally used in Ayurvedic medicine to treat diabetes. Gymnema is believed to help lower blood sugar levels by blocking the absorption of sugar in the intestines and increasing insulin production. Studies have shown that taking Gymnema supplements can help lower blood sugar levels in people with type 2 diabetes.

Bitter Melon is a fruit that is commonly used in traditional Chinese medicine to treat diabetes. Studies have shown that Bitter Melon can help lower blood sugar levels and improve insulin sensitivity. One study found that drinking bitter melon juice for four weeks resulted in lower fasting blood sugar levels and improved glucose tolerance in people with type 2 diabetes.

If you have diabetes, it's important to work with your healthcare provider to develop a comprehensive treatment plan and don't forget to monitor blood sugar levels regularly.

As mentioned earlier, there are also some lifestyle changes that can help manage diabetes. One of the most important lifestyle changes is to maintain a healthy diet. A diet that is high in fiber and low in sugar and carbohydrates can help regulate blood sugar levels and improve overall health.

Regular exercise is also helps to improve insulin sensitivity and can help lower blood sugar levels. Aim for at least 30 minutes of moderate-intensity exercise most days of the week.

Stress can also increase blood sugar levels and make it harder to manage the condition. Techniques such as meditation, deep breathing, and yoga can help reduce stress and improve overall health.

While there is no cure for diabetes, there are ways to manage the condition and prevent or delay complications and with the right approach, it is possible to live a healthy and fulfilling life.

dark circles under the eyes and bruising

ONE SPECIFIC AREA of interest is how certain herbs can help increase oxygen in the blood, which can help to reduce the appearance of dark circles and eye bags, and potentially reduce the risk of bruising. Let's explore the connection between oxygen levels in the blood and dark circles, and how herbal teas can help to increase oxygen in the bloodstream.

The skin around the eyes is thin and delicate, and it is not uncommon for people to develop dark circles and eye bags as they age. Dark circles can be caused by a number of factors, including genetics, lack of sleep, and poor nutrition. However, a lack of oxygen in the blood can also contribute to the appearance of dark circles. When the skin around the eyes is not getting enough oxygen, it can appear darker and more tired.

Ginkgo biloba and **Gotu kola** are both used to improve circulation and increase oxygen in the blood. Ginkgo is believed to work by dilating blood vessels, which allows for better blood flow and increased oxygen delivery to the skin while Gotu kola improves the elasticity of blood vessels, which in turn helps to improve blood flow. Both are rich in antioxidants, which can help to protect the skin from damage caused by free radicals.

Hawthorn is another popular herb that works by improving circulation and strengthening the walls of blood vessels, which in turn helps to improve the delivery of oxygen to the skin. Hawthorn is also believed to have a mild sedative effect, which can help to reduce stress and improve sleep, both of which can contribute to the appearance of dark circles.

To make a tea, simply add one or two teaspoons of dried herbs to a cup of boiling water. Let the tea steep for five to 10 minutes, then strain and drink. It is recommended to drink two to three cups of herbal tea per day to see the best results.

In addition to helping reduce the appearance of dark circles, increasing oxygen in the blood may also help to reduce the risk of bruising. Bruising occurs when blood vessels are damaged and blood leaks into the surrounding tissue, causing a discoloration of the skin.

A lack of oxygen in the blood can contribute to the formation of bruises, as it makes blood vessels more fragile and prone to breaking. By increasing the oxygen levels in the blood, herbs can help to improve the health and strength of blood vessels, reducing the risk of bruising.

diarrhea

Diarrhea has a number of causes, it is often caused by bacterial food poisoning, but it can also be caused by viruses and parasites found in drinking water. If you have food allergies such as lactose intolerance or coeliac disease, then eating the wrong meal could lead to diarrhea.

The first thing that you should do is focus on staying hydrated. Sports drinks are great because they can also balance electrolytes.

Before using herbal remedies to treat diarrhea, it is important to talk to your doctor first, as the cause of diarrhea may be worsened by certain herbs. Many herbs can also interact with any medication that you may be on, so make a doctor's appointment your first priority.

One of the best herbal remedies for diarrhea is **Carob powder**. This works by firming up your stool as it is high in fiber and can be taken as a tea.

Agrimony can be used in tea to treat diarrhea. It is a good source of tannins which can help stop diarrhea. However, it interacts with blood-thinning medication and some diabetes medication, so keep this in mind if you use either.

Taking **Blackberry leaf** tea can help to prevent diarrhea by drying up the mucous membranes of the intestine. Use one teaspoon mixed with boiling water to make a tea. This can also be done to a similar effect with **Raspberry leaf** tea.

Chamomile tea is good at reducing inflammation, which is helpful when treating diarrhea. Add Ginger to help digestion and a honey to taste.

If you have nowhere to be, then drinking your teas throughout the day will not only help reduce diarrhea but will also keep you hydrated throughout.

twenty-three
eyes

THERE ARE a variety of eye problems that people face, and herbal remedies can be a valuable tool for maintaining eye health and alleviating uncomfortable symptoms. From styes, to dry eye syndrome to glaucoma to cataracts to digital eye strain, there are herbs that can help support healthy vision and prevent damage to the eyes.

Styes

A sty in the eye, also known as a hordeolum, is typically caused by a bacterial infection of one of the oil glands in the eyelid. These glands are called meibomian glands and are responsible for producing oil that helps lubricate the eye.

When one of these glands becomes blocked or infected, it can cause a painful and swollen bump to form on the edge of the eyelid. The infection is usually caused by the bacterium Staphylococcus aureus, which is commonly found on the skin and can easily get into the oil glands.

Several factors can increase the likelihood of developing a sty in the eye, including poor hygiene, rubbing the eyes with dirty hands, using old or contaminated makeup, and wearing contact lenses for too long without properly cleaning them. Certain medical conditions such as blepharitis (inflammation of the eyelids) and rosacea (a skin condition that causes redness and bumps on the face) can also increase the risk of developing styes.

There are several herbal remedies that can help treat styes or horde-olums, depending on the specific condition. Here are some examples:

External hordeolum

This type of sty appears on the outer edge of the eyelid and is usually caused by an infection in the eyelash follicles.

A warm compress made with **Chamomile** tea, **Calendula** tea, or lavender tea can help soothe the affected area and encourage the sty to drain. Simply soak a clean cloth in the warm tea, wring out the excess liquid, and hold it gently against the affected eyelid for 10-15 minutes, several times a day.

Tea Tree Oil has natural antimicrobial properties that can help fight the bacteria causing the infection. Dilute a drop of tea tree oil in a teaspoon of carrier oil (such as coconut oil or olive oil), and apply it to the affected area with a cotton swab, taking care not to get it in the eye.

Internal hordeolum

This type of sty appears on the inner edge of the eyelid and is usually caused by an infection in the meibomian gland.

Like with external styes, a warm compress can help soothe the affected area and encourage drainage. You can use the same herbal teas as for external styes.

Eyebright is a natural astringent and anti-inflammatory herb that can help reduce swelling and pain. Make a tea with 1-2 teaspoons of dried eyebright in a cup of boiled water, let it cool, and use it as a warm compress on the affected eye. Don't use Eyebright if you have glaucoma.

<u>Recurrent hordeolum</u>

Some people may experience multiple styes in the same eye or in different eyes, which can be a sign of a chronic condition called meibomian gland dysfunction (MGD).

Omega-3s, found in flaxseed oil or fish oil, can help improve the quality of the oil produced by the meibomian glands and reduce inflammation in the eye. Take an omega-3 supplement daily or add more fatty fish to your diet.

Ginkgo Biloba is an herb that can help improve blood flow to the eye and reduce inflammation. Take a Ginkgo Biloba supplement daily or drink it as a tea.

Dry Eye Syndrome

First, let's talk about one of the most well-known eye problems: dry eye syndrome. Dry eye syndrome occurs when your eyes don't produce enough tears or when your tears evaporate too quickly. This can lead to uncomfortable symptoms like redness, itching, and a feeling like there's something in your eye. One effective herbal remedy for dry eye syndrome is **Omega-3 fatty acids** found in flaxseed oil or fish oil. These oils help to lubricate the eyes and reduce inflammation. They can be taken orally as a supplement or added to your diet in the form of fatty fish like salmon or mackerel, or they can also be applied topically to the eyelids to help lubricate the eyes and reduce inflammation.

Additionally, herbs like **Eyebright** and and **Fennel** can help to stimulate tear production and soothe irritated eyes. Eyebright can be taken as an herbal tea, in capsule form, or used as an eye wash. To make an eye wash, steep 1-2 teaspoons of dried eyebright in a cup of boiled water for 10-15 minutes, strain the liquid, and allow it to cool before using. Again, don't use Eyebright if you have glaucoma.

Fennel seeds can be chewed, brewed as an herbal tea, or used as an eye wash in the same way as eyebright.

Glaucoma

Another common eye problem is glaucoma. Glaucoma is a condition in which pressure builds up inside the eye, leading to damage of the optic nerve and potential vision loss. While there are no known herbal remedies that can cure glaucoma, there are some that may help to reduce pressure in the eyes.

One such herb is **Ginkgo Biloba**, which has been shown in some studies to improve blood flow to the eyes and reduce intraocular pressure.

Ginkgo Biloba can be taken orally as a supplement, brewed as a tea, or used in eye drops. Eye drops containing Ginkgo Biloba extract are available in some countries but are not approved for use in the United States. This is good reminder that people with glaucoma, or any other condition, should always work with their healthcare provider to monitor their condition and develop a comprehensive treatment plan.

Cataracts

Cataracts are another common eye problem that many people face as they age. Cataracts occur when the lens of the eye becomes cloudy, leading to blurry vision and potentially even vision loss. One herbal remedy that may help to prevent or slow the progression of cataracts is **Bilberry**.

Bilberry contains compounds called anthocyanins, which have been shown to help protect the eye from oxidative stress and improve blood flow.

In addition to Bilberry, other herbs that may be beneficial for eye health include **Marigold**, which is rich in lutein and zeaxanthin, two antioxidants that help to protect the eyes from damage, and **Ginseng**, which has been shown to improve visual function in people with glaucoma.

Bilberry and Marigold can be taken as a supplement in capsule form or used as an eye drop while Ginseng can be taken orally as a supplement or brewed as an herbal tea.

Some studies have also used Bilberry and Marigold extracts as an eye wash.

Digital Eye Strain

Finally, let's talk about one of the most common eye problems that many of us face on a daily basis: digital eye strain. With the rise of technology, more and more people are spending hours each day staring at screens, whether it's a computer, tablet, or smartphone. This can lead to symptoms like eye fatigue, dryness, and even headaches.

One herbal remedy that can help alleviate digital eye strain is **Chamomile**. Chamomile contains compounds which can help to reduce eye redness and irritation. Other herbs that may be helpful for digital eye strain include **Calendul**a, which is high in antioxidants that protect the eyes from oxidative stress, and **Lavender**, which has a calming effect that can help to reduce eye strain and promote relaxation.

Chamomile can be brewed as an herbal tea and used as a compress on the eyes. To make a chamomile compress, steep 1-2 teaspoons of dried chamomile flowers in a cup of boiled water for 10-15 minutes, strain the liquid, allow it to cool, soak a clean cloth or cotton ball in the tea, and apply it to closed eyes for 10-15 minutes.

Calendula and Lavender can be brewed as an herbal tea and used as a compress on the eyes in the same way as chamomile.

Alternatively, Lavender essential oil can be diluted with a carrier oil like coconut or olive oil and applied topically around the eyes (taking care to avoid getting it in the eyes).

twenty-four
fatigue

THERE ARE two types of fatigue, physical and mental. They often come together as a pair, but it is not uncommon to only suffer from one at a time. There are also different forms of physical fatigue (muscular fatigue vs. cardiovascular fatigue), but this is of little concern to herbal medicine and more of a sports science concern.

When it comes to fatigue, there is another way to categorize it. Short-term or acute fatigue as well as long-term or chronic fatigue.

Acute fatigue occurs after you have tired yourself out. Running a 10km race will lead to acute physical fatigue. Having a bad night's sleep could lead to acute physical and mental fatigue. Working for 10 hours straight can lead to acute mental fatigue.

Chronic fatigue is when you are feeling tired and lethargic all the time. Whether you have worked 10 hours or had three days of leisure.

Chronic fatigue is often caused by mental health conditions such as depression and anxiety. But insomnia is another common cause. Lifestyle factors can also lead to chronic fatigue because they can they disrupt your routine - an example would be going to bed much later than normal and not allowing your body and mind to rest fully.

An interesting cause of chronic fatigue is excessive exercise or dieting. People who go too far in their quest to lose weight can over-exert themselves in the gym and struggle to recover. Particularly if they are not consuming enough energy to sustain themselves.

The most well-researched herbal remedy for reducing fatigue is **Rhodiola Rosea**. It works really well for people who are physically and mentally tired after working incredibly hard. If you have been studying for 3 weeks for an exam, then rhodiola rosea is the herb for you.

Not only can it remove fatigue, but it can also increase cognition and focus. It is also a mood-boosting herb. You can either take it daily (50mg capsules) to avoid fatigue, or you can take it in response to fatigue (250-650mg).

Ashwagandha extract has been shown to reduce fatigue, but you need to be taking it daily to see the benefits. It is also very good for the treatment of depression and anxiety, both of which cause fatigue. This may be a good herbal remedy for chronic fatigue.

Coffee and **black tea** are good sources of caffeine, which is one of the most effective cures for physical fatigue. Though if you take caffeine too late in the day, it can affect sleep which affects fatigue. So be sensible with your usage.

Ayurveda promotes the use of **Coleus Forskohlii** for the treatment of low testosterone in men. Fatigue is one of the side effects of low testosterone that this herb can address. It is not effective for reducing fatigue in women. It should be taken in capsule form, with a dosage of 50mg per day being standard.

Turmeric appears to have a small effect on fatigue in people recovering from surgery. More research is required to see whether it can be effective in a more general sense. You can either supplement with curcumin tablets or use more turmeric in your food.

Traditional Chinese Medicine uses **Lingzi mushroom** to treat fatigue, depression, anxiety and to improve mood. It is only just starting to be looked at in Western medicine, but so far, the results look good. 5 grams of mushroom powder make a standard dose.

Panax Ginseng is also a popular herbal remedy, and it works well when drunk as tea.

twenty-five
fibromyalgia

FIBROMYALGIA IS a chronic condition that affects many people, particularly women. It is characterized by widespread pain throughout the body, as well as fatigue and a range of other symptoms. While the exact cause of fibromyalgia is not fully understood, it is believed to involve a combination of genetic, environmental, and lifestyle factors.

There is evidence to suggest that fibromyalgia is more common in women, and that the risk of developing the condition increases with age. While fibromyalgia can affect individuals of any age and gender, it has been reported to be more prevalent in women than men, with estimates ranging from 75% to 90% of people diagnosed with the condition being women.

There is also some evidence to suggest that menopause may be a risk factor for the development of fibromyalgia. Hormonal changes during menopause, such as decreases in estrogen levels, has been suggested as a possible factor and it is known to play a role in pain processing. If you are diagnosed with fibromyalgia check that this is not the result of disturbed sleep due to declining hormone levels during early peri menopause - this lack of sleep can lead to aches and pains as well as chronic fatigue, which all means that it will go away and it is not a long term condition. If you are early peri-menopausal it is better to do a blood test with a physician rather than an on-off-shelf test because the pin-prick test will not give an accurate reading of your fluctuating estrogen levels.

There has also been a study published in the Journal of Women's Health and it found that women who had gone through menopause were more likely to report symptoms of fibromyalgia than premenopausal women. The study did not establish a direct causal link between the two, and further research is needed to fully understand the relationship.

Symptoms of Fibromyalgia

The primary symptom of fibromyalgia is widespread pain throughout the body, which can be felt in the muscles, tendons, and ligaments.

This pain can be described as a deep, achy, or burning sensation that can be difficult to localize to one specific area of the body. In addition to pain, individuals may also experience fatigue, sleep disturbances, cognitive difficulties, and mood changes.

The fatigue can be severe and persistent, and may not improve with rest or sleep and sufferers may also experience sleep disturbances, such as difficulty falling or staying asleep, and may wake up feeling unrefreshed or still tired.

Cognitive difficulties, often referred to as "brain fog," is another symptom that can significantly impact daily functioning. It includes difficulty concentrating, memory problems, and difficulty processing information.

Mood changes, such as depression and anxiety, are also common and they can be related to the impact of the symptoms on daily life, as well as the underlying changes in the brain and nervous system that contribute to fibromyalgia.

Other symptoms include migraines and tension headaches and digestive issues such as bloating, constipation IBS).

Interestingly, many, if not all, of these symptoms can be caused by the menopause.

Diagnosis

Diagnosing fibromyalgia can be challenging because the symptoms are often non-specific and can be similar to those of other medical conditions. There is no definitive test for fibromyalgia, and the diagnosis is typically made based on a combination of clinical evaluation, medical history, and exclusion of other conditions.

The American College of Rheumatology (ACR) has developed diagnostic criteria for fibromyalgia, which includes widespread pain and tenderness in at least 11 of 18 specific tender points on the body, as well as a history of widespread pain lasting for at least three months.

The 18 tender points are located at:

1. Occiput (back of the head)
2. Low cervical spine (base of the neck)
3. Trapezius muscle (shoulder blade region)
4. Supraspinatus muscle (shoulder region)
5. Second rib (upper chest)
6. Lateral epicondyle (outer elbow)
7. Gluteal region (buttocks)
8. Greater trochanter (hip)
9. Knee (medial fat pad)

In addition, the diagnosis may also involve ruling out other medical conditions that can cause similar symptoms, such as thyroid disorders, rheumatoid arthritis, and lupus.

Causes

While the exact cause of fibromyalgia is not fully understood, genetic studies have shown that it tends to run in families, which suggests that there may be a genetic component to the condition. Researchers are currently working to identify specific genes that may be involved.

Some experts believe it may be caused by an abnormality in the way the brain and nervous system process pain signals. This theory is supported by the fact that people with fibromyalgia often experience pain in response to stimuli that would not typically be considered painful, such as light touch or mild pressure.

Exposure to certain environmental factors, such as traumatic events, infections, or chronic stress, is also believed to increase a person's risk of developing fibromyalgia while poor sleep habits, a lack of physical activity, and a diet high in processed foods are all thought to be possible contributors.

Herbal Treatment for Fibromyalgia

Fortunately, there are several herbal remedies that can help manage the symptoms of fibromyalgia. Here are some of the best herbs for each cause of fibromyalgia:

Genetic predisposition: While there is no herb that can cure genetic predisposition, there are several herbs that can help manage the symptoms. **St. John's Wort** is a popular herb for treating depression, a common symptom of fibromyalgia. Other herbs that may be beneficial include **Skullcap, Passionflower**, and **Valerian root**.

Environmental factors: **Milk Thistle** is a powerful herb that can help support liver function and aid in detoxification. Other herbs include **Dandelion root, Burdock root**, and **Nettle**.

Hormonal imbalances: **Black Cohosh** is often used to manage menopausal symptoms, and may also be helpful for managing fibromyalgia symptoms related to hormonal imbalances. Other herbs that may be help include **Dong Quai, Red Clover**, and **Chasteberry**.

Chronic stress: **Ashwagandha** is a powerful adaptogenic herb that can help the body cope with stress. Other herbs include **Holy Basil, Rhodiola**, and **Eleuthero**.

Physical trauma: **Arnica** is a great herb for managing pain and inflammation associated with physical trauma. Other herbs include **Turmeric, Ginger**, and **Devil's Claw**.

If you want to use a herbal tea, you can try the following soothing tea that can help manage fibromyalgia symptoms:

Ingredients:

- 1 teaspoon chamomile flowers
- 1 teaspoon skullcap

- 1 teaspoon lemon balm
- 1 teaspoon St. John's Wort

Directions:

1. Combine herbs in a tea infuser or tea ball.
2. Place infuser or tea ball in a cup.
3. Pour boiling water over the herbs.
4. Cover and let steep for 10-15 minutes.
5. Strain and enjoy.

twenty-six
fever

FEVERS ARE one of the most common symptoms that people experience, and they can be caused by a wide range of factors, from infections to heat exhaustion. In this chapter, I'll walk you through some of the most common types of fevers, what causes them, and the best herbal remedies to treat them.

Let's start with the most common type of fever: the viral fever. As the name suggests, viral fevers are caused by viruses, and they can range from mild to severe. The common cold and flu are both examples of viral fevers. To treat a viral fever, I recommend using herbs that have antiviral properties, such as **Echinacea**, **Elderberry**, and **Garlic**. These herbs can help to boost your immune system and fight off the virus causing the fever.

Next up, we have bacterial fevers. These are caused by bacterial infections, such as strep throat or urinary tract infections. To treat a bacterial fever, you'll need to use herbs that have antibacterial properties. Some great options include **Oregano**, **Thyme**, and **Tea Tree** oil. These herbs can help to kill the bacteria causing the fever and reduce inflammation in the body.

Another type of fever is the fungal fever, which is caused by fungal infections like ringworm or candidiasis. For this type of fever, I recommend using herbs that have antifungal properties, such as **Pau d'arco**, **Garlic**, and **Oregano**. These herbs can help to kill the fungi causing the fever and improve your overall immune system.

Sometimes, fevers can also be caused by heat exhaustion or dehydration. In these cases, it's important to stay hydrated and cool down your body. Some great herbs for this purpose include Peppermint, Chamomile, and Lemon Balm. These herbs can help to reduce inflammation and soothe your body.

In addition to these types of fevers, there are also chronic fevers that last for an extended period of time, often with no clear cause. These fevers can be a sign of an underlying medical condition, such as an autoimmune disorder or cancer. If you're experiencing a chronic fever, it's important to see a healthcare professional to determine the underlying cause. That being said, there are still some herbal remedies that may be helpful in managing the symptoms of a chronic fever. Some good options include **Ginseng**, **Ashwagandha**, and **Licorice** root, which can help to support your immune system and reduce inflammation.

There are many different types of fevers, each with their own unique causes and treatments. Whether you're dealing with a viral, bacterial, fungal, or chronic fever, there are a variety of herbal remedies that can help to reduce inflammation, boost your immune system, and fight off the underlying cause of the fever. As always, it's important to speak with a healthcare professional before starting any new herbal remedies, particularly if you're dealing with a chronic or severe fever.

twenty-seven
gout

GOUT IS a type of arthritis that occurs when there's a buildup of uric acid in the body. This uric acid buildup can lead to the formation of sharp crystals in the joints, causing inflammation and intense pain.

Uric acid is formed from the breakdown of purines, which can be produced naturally in the body or found in many foods, including red meat, seafood, and alcohol.

When the body breaks down purines, it produces uric acid. Having a regular production of uric acid has no side effects, and your body is pretty good at eliminating it via your urine. However, too much uric acid leads to the inflammation in the joints. When this happens, you are diagnosed as having gout.

Another factor that can contribute to gout is genetics. Some people are simply more prone to developing gout due to genetic factors that affect the way their body processes uric acid. Other risk factors include obesity, high blood pressure, and certain medical conditions such as kidney disease or diabetes.

The good news is that there are a number of herbal remedies that can help to manage the symptoms of gout and reduce the risk of future flare-ups.

The most well-researched herbal remedy for gout is **Tart Cherry juice**. The idea is that the tart cherry juice can remove the uric acid from the bloodstream, rather than only targeting the inflammation.

However, the results so far are mixed. This may work well in combination with other ingredients such as ginger.

Other herbs that may be helpful include Turmeric, and Devil's Claw.

It's also important to make lifestyle changes to manage gout, such as maintaining a healthy weight, drinking plenty of water, and avoiding foods that are high in purines. By taking a holistic approach to managing gout, including incorporating herbal remedies, you can help to reduce inflammation, manage pain, and improve your overall quality of life.

There are also many herbal remedies for reducing inflammation, and some of them are particularly good at treating gout.

Ginger poultices can be effective (applied to the joints that hurt) or drinking ginger tea.

Stinging nettle tea can also and **Dandelion tea** is also a well-known herbal remedy for joint pain.

Traditional Chinese Medicine has a vast number of herbal remedies for gout. **Jiawei Simiao** powder and cream are very popular.

twenty-eight
grief

THERE IS no herb that can make grief better but there are some that can ease anxiety, and help you to relax by encouraging calmness.

Chamomile has a natural calming effect and both Chamomile and **Lavender** can calm and help sleep.

Other teas to consider if Lavender and Chamomile are not working for you include **Lemon Balm** and **Valerian root**. Leave the Valerian root to stew for up to 15 minutes.

All teas can be taken several times a day but if you are on any other medications it is always better to check with your doctor.

hair health and growth

ALONGSIDE SKIN, your hair is another crucial part of your integumentary system. It plays a crucial rule in skin maintenance, helps keep us warm, and protects us from the environment.

The health of your hair is also tied in to your overall health, and good hair maintenance can have other benefits in the long term.

Ayurveda, TCM, and Native American medicine all believe that hair problems are connected to kidney health and although hair loss can be a sign of kidney failure, but there are many non-kidney-related reasons why you may be losing hair or prematurely becoming grey. Age, stress, and diet are often they main causes.

In this section we will be looking at two areas of importance: hair growth and hair colour.

Hair Growth

Interestingly, there are a lot of herbal remedies, particularly in Native American medicine, that are designed to deal with hair growth.

Saw Palmetto is used for both hair and skincare. It is believed to work through balancing hormones. While it can help men grow their hair, it may have the opposite effect on women. Native American women use it to remove facial hair.

Essential oils such as **Lavender**, **Rosemary**, and **Thyme** have been used historically to encourage hair growth. Rubbing them into your hair before bed can not only help stimulate hair growth but can also relax you and help you sleep better.

Green tea has been shown to help prevent baldness in both men and women. Green tea that has a high concentration of epigallocatechin (EGCG) has been shown to be particularly effective. You can either drink it or take it in capsule form.

Recipe: To make the Rosemary tincture add 6 tbsp dry or fresh rosemary to 60ml of apple cider vinegar (4 tbsp). Let it steep for at least 20 minutes. Wash and dry hair (don't use conditioner) and then, using a cotton wool bud, dab the mixture onto your scalp and massage it gently. Leave it for 10 minutes then wash hair again as normal. epeat this process around twice a week.

Rosemary has vitamins B6, B2, A and C as well as iron, magnesium, phosphorus, zinc, calcium and other antioxidants and this why it is thought to be especially good for hair and scalp health. Repeat this process around twice a week. The apple cider vinegar cleanses the scalp and add shine to your hair.

Don't forget to dab a little of the mixture onto your arm first to make sure you don't have a negative reaction to it.

Hair Colour

Your hair turning grey is a natural part of growing older. Our hair goes through growth and regrowth cycles all the time, with new follicles replacing old ones. Once we reach middle age, our new follicles begin to come out white or grey rather than our natural color.

But it isn't just aging; stress and lifestyle factors can also affect your hair color. The idea that stress or grief can turn your hair grey is not a myth!

Ayurvedic medicine teaches that **Coconut oil** applied to the hair can help to prevent greying as you age. **Black tea** used topically may also be able to help.

Traditional Chinese Medicine recommends using the flowering plant **Fo-Ti** (also known as Tuber fleeceflower). 1000mg twice per day. However, overconsumption can affect liver health, so be careful when using it.

An **oil extract of rosemary** may effectively prevent grey hair; as with coconut oil, you should apply it to your hair for several weeks.

Finding ways to reduce stress and anxiety and treat insomnia may help prevent your hair from turning white or grey. A diet filled with nutrients is also very effective.

Sage, Nettle, Peppermint, Chamolile (as well as Rosemary) are all used (and can be taken as a tea) to help dandruff. My favorite for hair is always Rosemary,

Greasy Hair

As a herbalist, I have encountered many people who struggle with greasy hair. It can be frustrating, embarrassing, and even affect self-esteem.

Overproduction of sebum

The most common cause of greasy hair is an overproduction of sebum, which is the natural oil produced by the sebaceous glands in the scalp. It is this which can make the hair look oily and greasy. This can be caused by hormonal imbalances, genetics, or even stress.

Herbs that can help regulate the production of sebum include **Rosemary**, **Sage**, and **Lavender**. Rosemary has antimicrobial and anti-inflammatory properties that can help reduce scalp inflammation, while sage has astringent properties that can help tighten the pores on the scalp. Lavender has a calming effect on the scalp and can help reduce stress, which can contribute to an overproduction of sebum.

Recipe: Mix equal parts rosemary, sage, and lavender in a bowl. Boil 2 cups of water and add the herbs. Cover and let steep for 30 minutes. Strain and use as a rinse after shampooing. Do not use if pregnant or breastfeeding.

Hair products

The pH of the scalp is naturally acidic, with a pH between 4.5 and 5.5. Using hair products that are too alkaline can disrupt this balance and cause the sebaceous glands to produce more oil.

It means that using hair products that are too harsh or contain too many chemicals can strip the hair of its natural oils, causing the scalp to overcompensate by producing more oil and this can lead to greasy hair and even dandruff.

Herbs that can help soothe an irritated scalp and restore the natural pH balance include **Chamomile**, **Calendula**, and **Aloe Vera**. Chamomile has anti-inflammatory properties that can help reduce scalp irritation, while calendula has antiseptic properties that can help fight against fungal and bacterial infections. Aloe vera has a cooling effect on the scalp and can help soothe inflammation.

Recipe: Mix equal parts chamomile, calendula, and aloe vera gel in a bowl. Apply to the scalp and hair, and leave on for 15-20 minutes before rinsing off with water. Do not use if allergic to ragweed or related plants.

Diet

Eating a diet that is high in processed foods, sugar, and unhealthy fats can also cause the sebaceous glands to produce more oil than necessary.

Herbs that can help balance the sebaceous glands and promote healthy hair growth include **Nettle**, **Horsetail**, and **Burdock root**. Nettle has astringent properties that can help regulate the production of sebum, while horsetail is rich in silica, which can help strengthen hair follicles. Burdock root has anti-inflammatory properties that can help reduce scalp inflammation.

Nettle is also a natural diuretic that can help reduce water retention and bloating.

Recipe: Mix equal parts nettle, horsetail, and burdock root in a bowl. Boil 2 cups of water and add the herbs. Cover and let steep for 30 minutes. Strain and use as a rinse after shampooing. Do not use if pregnant or breastfeeding

Stress

You may be surprised to realise that stress can also contribute to an overproduction of sebum. It increases the levels of androgens in the body, which can stimulate the sebaceous glands to produce more oil.

This is why stress management techniques like meditation and yoga can be helpful in reducing the symptoms of greasy hair.

Dandruff

Dandruff is a common scalp condition that affects millions of people worldwide. It is characterized by flaking and itching of the scalp, which can be both uncomfortable and embarrassing. While there are many causes of dandruff, the good news is that it can be effectively treated with herbal remedies.

Dandruff can be caused by a variety of factors such as dry scalp, fungal infections, poor diet, and stress.

Dry scalp can be caused by a lack of moisture in the skin, which can be exacerbated by cold weather, low humidity, or harsh shampoos.

Aloe vera is a popular remedy for dry scalp due to its natural moisturizing properties. Aloe vera gel can be applied to the scalp and left on for 30 minutes before rinsing off.

Rosemary is another herb that has been used for centuries to treat dandruff and promote hair growth. It contains antioxidants that can soothe a dry and itchy scalp.

Rosemary leaves can be boiled in water and used as a rinse after shampooing. **Jojoba oil** is another natural moisturizer that can be massaged into the scalp and left on for 30 minutes before washing off. It contains vitamin E and antioxidants that can promote healthy hair growth.

Fungal infections can also cause dandruff by feeding on the oils secreted by the scalp. **Tea tree oil** is a natural antifungal that can help kill the Malassezia fungus that causes dandruff. It also has anti-inflammatory properties that can soothe an itchy scalp. A few drops of tea tree oil can be mixed with shampoo and massaged into the scalp.

Neem is another herb with antifungal and antibacterial properties that can help kill the fungus that causes dandruff.

Neem leaves can be boiled in water and used as a rinse after shampooing. **Eucalyptus** is also known for its natural antifungal properties and can be used in the same manner as rosemary and neem.

A poor diet that is low in essential nutrients, particularly zinc and B vitamins, can also contribute to dandruff. **Burdock root** is rich in zinc and can help nourish the scalp and promote healthy hair growth.

Burdock root can be boiled in water and used as a rinse after shampooing. Ginger is also a natural anti-inflammatory that can soothe an inflamed scalp (and promote hair growth). Ginger can be grated and mixed with warm coconut oil before being applied to the scalp and left on for 30 minutes before washing off.

thirty
headaches &
migraines

HEADACHES CAN HAVE many different causes. Stress, dehydration, issues with eyesight, too much alcohol the night before, or they can be caused by colds or the flu.

They may also be caused by a head injury, or they could be indicative of something more serious, so keep this in mind if they last for several days or are accompanied by other symptoms.

The first herbal remedy to look at when trying to cure a headache or migraine has to be **Lavender**. This plant has been used to treat headaches for thousands of years. Making a compress with dried lavender and resting it on your forehead is quite effective, as is using essential oils in a diffuser or in a bowl of water.

Interestingly, **Peppermint** appears to have the most scientific evidence of being an effective cure for headaches. Two studies have found that Peppermint oil can significantly reduce the severity of a tension headache within 15 minutes.

African Geranium is effective at treating headaches and migraines that are associated with acute bronchitis. But they don't seem to do much outside of this area. If your headache is the result of a chesty cough, then this may be the plant for you. A tincture of the root extract is the preferred method to take it.

Native American medicine uses **Osha**, also known as Bear Root, to treat headaches. It can be used in teas or poultices. It can also be chewed. **Ginger** also appears to be quite helpful in treating headaches and is popular in Traditional Chinese Medicine.

The Ancient Greeks used **Feverfew** to treat headaches, and this is still the case in modern Greece, the Balkans, and many Eastern European countries.

Most herbal teas should help because they can provide hydration, or they can help to reduce stress and anxiety. Both dehydration and stress are common causes of headaches.

thirty-one
hives

IF YOU'RE DEALING with hives, you're not alone. These raised, itchy bumps can be caused by a number of things, from an allergic reaction to stress. Luckily, there are plenty of herbal remedies that can help you find relief. Allergies, skin conditions (itchy skin) and stress are covered in other chapters so take a look at these as well as the information below.

First off, it's important to understand that not all hives are created equal. There are two main types of hives: acute and chronic. Acute hives usually last less than six weeks and are often caused by an allergic reaction to something like food, medication, or insect bites. Chronic hives, on the other hand, last longer than six weeks and can be caused by things including autoimmune disorders, stress, and infections.

No matter what type of hives you have, they can be a real pain to deal with. Here are some of the most common problems associated with hives, as well as some herbal remedies that can help.

Problem: Itching

Hives are notoriously itchy, which can be incredibly frustrating, and scratching can make the itching worse and even lead to infections.

Solution: Aloe vera

Aloe vera is a well-known natural remedy for skin irritation, including itching. Apply some aloe vera gel to the affected area to soothe the itching and reduce inflammation. You can also try adding a few drops of peppermint oil to your aloe vera gel for an extra cooling effect.

Problem: Swelling

Hives can cause swelling in the affected area, which can be uncomfortable and even make it difficult to move.

Solution: Chamomile

Chamomile is a natural anti-inflammatory that can help reduce swelling. You can make a chamomile tea and soak a cloth in it, then apply the cloth to the affected area. You can also apply chamomile essential oil to the affected area, but be sure to dilute it with a carrier oil first.

Problem: Redness

Hives can cause redness in the affected area, which can be unsightly and make you feel self-conscious.

Solution: Calendula

Calendula is a natural anti-inflammatory and antiseptic that can help reduce redness and prevent infection. You can apply calendula oil or salve to the affected area to help soothe the skin.

Problem: Stress

Stress can exacerbate hives and make them worse.

Solution: Lemon balm

Lemon balm is a natural sedative that can help reduce stress and anxiety. You can make a lemon balm tea and drink it to help calm your nerves. You can also apply lemon balm essential oil to the affected area to help soothe the skin.

Problem: Allergic reaction

If your hives are caused by an allergic reaction, you need to identify and avoid the allergen.

Solution: Nettle

Nettle is a natural antihistamine that can help reduce allergic reactions. You can make a nettle tea and drink it to help reduce your symptoms. You can also apply nettle cream or ointment to the affected area to help soothe the skin.

In addition to these herbal remedies, there are some other things you can do to help manage your hives.

As tempting as it may be, scratching can make your hives worse and even lead to infections. Take a cool bath, it can help soothe your skin and reduce itching and inflammation.

Tight clothing can rub against your hives and make them worse so try to stick to loose, breathable clothing to help keep your skin cool and comfortable.

thirty-two
immune system

WHEN IT COMES to your immune system, there are a lot of misconceptions. Most people are not sure what constitutes an immune system and what its role is exactly.

Your immune system involves your skin, hair, eyelashes, mucus, stomach acid, and mucus membranes. These make up your innate immune system and work like a security team. They want to know what is trying to get into your system and whether they are friendly or not.

Your innate immune system works immediately and is a little scattergun in its approach. There can be friendly fire. Your adaptive immune system is more ponderous. It aims to recognize what is in your system and fight known infections.

The ultimate goal for an immune system is not to make it all-powerful but for it to be functioning correctly. An overpowered immune system can lead to autoimmune diseases, where the immune system begins to attack healthy cells in your body.

You only want to boost your immune system if your immune system is currently in a weakened state.

But there are many causes of weakened immune systems:

- Age
- Lifestyle choices
- Disease
- Genetics

Finding herbal remedies to boost your immune system should come alongside lifestyle changes such as improving your diet, sleeping more, managing stress, and exercising regularly.

In Ayurveda, people eat bitter foods to protect their immune system when sick. The idea is that when animals get sick in nature, they tend to chew on more bitter plants than usual.

Foods such as cruciferous vegetables, **Green tea**, **Coffee**, and **Citrus Peel**, are all supposed to help strengthen your immune system.

Honey may be helpful in boosting your immune system, as are **Chamomile**, **Cinnamon**, **Ginger**, and **Cardamom seeds**. Making teas or recipes with these ingredients may offer some protection.

There is some evidence that **Stinging Nettles** can be effective at boosting your immune system. You can either use 300 mg twice per day of frozen leaf or you can make tea from the leaves.

Tulbaghia Violacea is an African herb that is used to fight off infection. There is some scientific backing to these claims as well. Traditional Chinese Medicine uses **Thunder God Vine** for the immune system. This is best taken in capsule form.

Another herb that is getting quite a lot of attention is the Tibetan herb **Oxytropis Falcate**, also known as the King of Herbs.

Elderberry is used as a remedy for viral infections like the flu and common cold. It stimulates the circulation, causing sweating which effectively cleanses the body.

Elderberry syrup is the common delivery method and 1-3 tablespoons can be taken per day during infection.

thirty-three
inflammation

WHEN YOU GET INJURED or sick, your immune system springs into action and attempts to kill any infection and/or begin the process of healing. This is a good thing and should be encouraged. But too much inflammation can exacerbate problems. Inflammation that lasts for too long can lead to diseases or injury.

Luckily, herbal medicine is really good at treating inflammation. Here are a number of herbal remedies that you can use to treat inflammation:

Studies have found that 2 grams of **Ginger** made into a tea can help to reduce inflammation. **Turmeric** is also very effective at treating inflammation.

An interesting treatment for inflammation is to use every gardener's worst nightmare **Japanese Knotweed**. A 2010 study found that a supplement containing 200 mg of Japanese Knotweed led to a 25% decrease in inflammation.

Panax Ginseng appears to be slightly effective, as does **Stinging Nettle** tea. **Cannabis** is being very closely looked at for its anti-inflammatory properties. Medical marijuana is continuing to astound the medical community at its many benefits.

Witch Hazel is well known for helping with many types of inflammation. Indigenous to North America, the bark aqueous infusion was used in aboriginal medicine to treat haemorrhages, inflammations and haemorrhoids. According the other European Medicines Agency (Assessment report on Hamamelis Virginiana L. Cortex, 2009) there is some evidence for the effectiveness of Witch Hazel. It is used as an astringent and anti-inflammatory product for the treatment of minor skin injuries, local inflammation of skin and mucous membranes; for bruises and localized inflamed swellings; to treat vascular disorders including hemorrhoids, varicose veins, phlebitis and other conditions associated with poor venous tone or congestion; menorrhagia and metrorrhagia; diarrhea; as a protective against oxidative stress and ultraviolet radiation.

One of the best ways to treat chronic inflammation is to look at improving lifestyle factors. Sleeping more, exercising more, eating a healthy diet such as the Mediterranean diet, and most importantly of all, prioritizing your mental health.

As always, herbal medicine can help with all of this. Particularly the sleep and mental health side of things. Though there are many herbal remedies that can improve your nutritional health and your exercise performance.

Inflammation can be seen as the route cause of most chronic illnesses, but you have to go further back than that. What causes inflammation? Stress, smoking, insomnia, weight gain, a lack of nutrients in your diet? Address these issues, and you are well on your way to living a life without chronic inflammation and its resulting illnesses.

thirty-four
irritable bowel syndrome (ibs)

IRRITABLE BOWEL SYNDROME (IBS) can be a challenging condition to manage, and it affects millions of people worldwide. IBS can cause a range of symptoms, including abdominal pain, bloating, constipation, and diarrhea, and it is caused by various factors.

IBS is a complex condition with many potential causes, and understanding the underlying mechanisms can help people manage their symptoms more effectively.

One of the potential causes of IBS is an imbalance in the gut microbiome, which, as we have seen, is the collection of microorganisms that live in the digestive tract. Research suggests that alterations in the gut microbiome can lead to inflammation and changes in the digestive system that may contribute to symptoms such as abdominal pain, bloating, and diarrhea. Some research suggests that taking probiotics, which are supplements containing beneficial bacteria, may help to rebalance the gut microbiome and improve IBS symptoms in some people. To this end, the probiotic strain Bifidobacterium infantis has been found to be particularly effective for those with gut microbiome imbalances.

Food sensitivities are another potential cause of IBS. Dairy products, for example, contain lactose, which some people have difficulty digesting. Gluten, a protein found in wheat, barley, and rye, may trigger symptoms in people with celiac disease or non-celiac gluten sensitivity while FODMAPs, a type of carbohydrate found in many foods, can be difficult for some people to digest and can contribute to IBS. You will want to try and identify trigger foods so that you can avoid them which can be a very effective way to manage the condition.

Stress can also play a role in the development of IBS. When the body is under stress, it releases hormones that can impact the digestive system, leading to abdominal pain and diarrhea. Stress reduction techniques, such as meditation, yoga, and deep breathing exercises, can be help.

Abnormal muscular contractions in the digestive system can also contribute to IBS. The muscles in the digestive system may contract too much or too little, leading to symptoms such as abdominal pain, constipation, and diarrhea. Herbs that help to regulate these contractions, such as antispasmodics, can help with this condition.

Finally, abnormalities in the nervous system can be the cause. The digestive system is regulated by the enteric nervous system, which communicates with the central nervous system. Disruptions in this communication can cause IBS symptoms. In this case, you would look to herbs that can act as antidepressants and reduce anxiety to help regulate the nervous system.

While the exact cause of IBS is not fully understood, it is likely that multiple factors contribute to its development . Addressing the underlying causes of IBS, such as gut microbiome imbalances, food sensitivities, stress, abnormal muscular contractions, and nervous system abnormalities, can all help to improve your quality of life.

The good news is that several herbs can help manage the different causes of IBS. Let's explore some of the best herbal remedies for IBS.

One of the most effective herbs for managing stress and IBS is **Chamomile** which, as well as reducing inflammation, calms the nervous system. Other herbs that can help include Lavender and Lemon Balm. For chamomile tea you can drink up to 3 cups a day.

Peppermint is a great solution for managing food sensitivities. It can help relax the muscles in the digestive system as well as reducing inflammation. While Peppermint is often taken as a tea, Peppermint oil capsules can be particularly effective for abdominal pain and bloating. Other herbs that can help with food sensitivities include Fennel and Ginger.

Licorice root can help manage gut microbiome imbalances and IBS. It contains compounds that can support the growth of beneficial gut bacteria and reduces inflammation. Marshmallow root is also great for the gut microbiome.

To make a Licorice root tea, add one teaspoon of dried licorice root to a cup of boiling water. Cover the cup and let it steep for ten minutes. Strain and drink up to three cups of licorice tea daily.

Finally, if the cause is inflammation, then there are many inflammatory-fighting herbs one of which is **Turmeric** that not only can help reduce inflammation in the gut but also improve digestion.

To make a Turmeric tea, add one teaspoon of ground turmeric to a cup of boiling water. Cover the cup and let it steep for ten minutes. Add a pinch of black pepper and a teaspoon of honey to taste.

If you have IBS then try to avoid Senna, Rhubarb root and Buckthorn bark tea which, although generally good for the digestive system, are all natural laxatives that can cause cramping, bloating, and diarrhea, and can worsen IBS symptoms.

thirty-five
insect bites

INSECT BITES CAN BE a real pain, both literally and figuratively. And while they might seem like an inevitable part of summertime, there are actually some easy herbal remedies you can use to help soothe and heal those bites. But before we get into the remedies themselves, it's important to understand that not all insect bites are created equal. Here are some of the most common types of insect bites, and what you need to know about each one.

First up, we've got mosquito bites. These are probably the most common type of insect bite, and chances are you've got a few of them right now. Mosquito bites can cause a lot of itching and swelling, which can be really frustrating.

Mosquito Bites

Mosquito bites are one of the most common types of insect bites, and they can be very itchy and irritating. Mosquitoes are attracted to warm, moist areas of the body, so they tend to bite around the ankles, wrists, and neck. Some people may experience a more severe reaction to mosquito bites, with redness, swelling, and even blistering.

One of the best herbal remedies for mosquito bites is **Chamomile**. This soothing herb can help reduce inflammation and calm the skin, providing relief from the itching and irritation of mosquito bites. To use Chamomile for mosquito bites, steep a tea bag in hot water for a few minutes, then let it cool down. Place the tea bag on the affected area and hold it there for a few minutes.

Another effective herbal remedy for mosquito bites is **Lavender**. This fragrant herb has natural antiseptic and anti-inflammatory properties, which can help reduce the swelling and redness of the bites. You can apply Lavender essential oil directly to the bite, or mix a few drops of the oil with a carrier oil like coconut or olive oil and apply the mixture to the affected area.

A third option for treating mosquito bites is **Aloe Vera**. This cooling plant can help reduce inflammation and itching, while also providing a protective barrier to prevent further irritation. Simply break off a leaf of the aloe vera plant and apply the gel to the bite.

Bee Stings

Next, we've got bee stings. These are a bit more serious than mosquito bites. Bee stings can be painful and even dangerous for people who are allergic to bees. When a bee stings, it injects venom into the skin, causing pain, swelling, and redness and some people may also experience a severe allergic reaction, with symptoms like difficulty breathing, hives, and swelling of the face and throat. If you've been stung by a bee and you're having trouble breathing or experiencing other symptoms, seek medical attention right away.

But if your bee sting is relatively mild, there are a few herbal remedies you can use to help soothe the pain and reduce swelling.

One of the best herbal remedies for bee stings is **Plantain**. This common weed has natural anti-inflammatory properties, and it can help reduce the pain and swelling of bee stings. To use Plantain for bee stings, crush a fresh plantain leaf and apply it directly to the affected area. You can also make a poultice by mashing the leaves and applying them to the skin with a bandage or cloth.

Another effective herbal remedy for bee stings is **Basil**. This fragrant herb contains natural compounds that can help reduce inflammation and pain. To use basil for bee stings, crush a few fresh leaves and apply them to the bite, or mix the crushed leaves with a carrier oil like olive or coconut oil and apply the mixture to the affected area.

A third option for treating bee stings is **Thyme**. This flavorful herb has natural antiseptic and anti-inflammatory properties, which can help reduce swelling and pain. To use thyme, steep a handful of fresh thyme leaves in hot water for a few minutes, then let the mixture cool. Apply the thyme-infused water to the affected area with a clean cloth or cotton ball.

Tick Bites

Ticks are another common insect that can leave a nasty bite. Not only are tick bites itchy and irritating, but ticks are tiny arachnids that can transmit diseases like Lyme disease and Rocky Mountain spotted fever. When a tick bites, it burrows into the skin and feeds on blood. Some people may not notice a tick bite right away, but symptoms can include redness, itching, and a bullseye-shaped rash.

If you've been bitten by a tick, it's important to remove it as soon as possible. You can do this with a pair of tweezers by grasping the tick as close to the skin as possible and pulling it straight out. After you've removed the tick, wash the bite with soap and water and keep an eye on it for any signs of infection. Once you have washed the area then you can try some of these remedies.

One of the best herbal remedies for tick bites is **Tea Tree** oil. This powerful essential oil has natural antiseptic and anti-inflammatory properties, which can help reduce the risk of infection and calm the skin. To use tea tree oil for tick bites, mix a few drops of the oil with a carrier oil like coconut or olive oil, and apply the mixture to the affected area.

Another effective herbal remedy for tick bites is **Eucalyptus**. This fragrant herb has natural anti-inflammatory and pain-relieving properties, which can help reduce the swelling and discomfort of tick bites. Mix a few drops of Eucalyptus essential oil with a carrier oil (olive or coconut oil) and apply the mixture to the affected area.

A third option for treating tick bites is **Rosemary**. This fragrant herb has natural antiseptic and anti-inflammatory properties, which can help reduce the risk of infection and calm the skin. To use rosemary steep a handful of fresh rosemary leaves in hot water for a few minutes, then let the mixture cool. Apply the rosemary-infused water to the affected area with a clean cloth or cotton ball.

Spider Bites

Finally, we've got spider bites. While most spiders aren't harmful to humans, spider bites can range from minor to very serious, depending on the type of spider and the person's reaction. Some spider bites can cause redness, swelling, and pain, while others can cause fever, muscle spasms, and even death.

If you think you've been bitten by a spider and you're experiencing symptoms like difficulty breathing, nausea, or severe pain, seek medical attention immediately.

But if your spider bite is relatively mild, there are a few herbal remedies you can use to help reduce pain and inflammation.

Calendulas bright yellow flower has natural anti-inflammatory and wound-healing properties, which can help reduce the redness and swelling of spider bites and promote healing. To use calendula for spider bites, crush a few fresh flowers and apply the juice directly to the affected area, or make a poultice by mashing the flowers and applying them to the skin with a bandage or cloth.

Another effective herb is **Witch Hazel**. This astringent herb can help reduce inflammation and pain, while also promoting healing. Simply apply a few drops of Witch Hazel to a cotton ball and apply it to the affected area.

A third option for is **Turmeric**. This brightly colored spice has natural anti-inflammatory and pain-relieving properties, which can help reduce the redness and discomfort of spider bites. To use Turmeric, mix a teaspoon of turmeric powder with a little water to make a paste, and apply the paste to the affected area.

You can also try **Chamomile** tea. Simply brew a cup of chamomile tea and let it cool. Then, apply the tea bag directly to the bite. The chamomile will help soothe the pain and reduce inflammation.

Fire Ant Bite

Fire ant bites can be particularly painful, and they can also cause a lot of itching and swelling. If you've ever been bitten by a fire ant, you know how uncomfortable it can be. One of the best herbal remedies for fire ant bites is **Witch Hazel**. This astringent plant can help reduce swelling and inflammation, and it can also provide some relief from the itching. To use Witch Hazel, soak a cotton ball or a clean cloth in Witch Hazel and apply it to the affected area. You can also pour some witch hazel into a spray bottle and spray it directly onto the bite.

Another great herbal remedy for fire ant bites is **Calendula**, with its anti-inflammatory properties it can help reduce the redness and swelling associated with insect bites. To use calendula for fire ant bites, you can make a simple salve. Start by melting some beeswax in a double boiler, then add some calendula-infused oil (you can make this by steeping dried calendula flowers in oil for several weeks). Stir the mixture until the wax is fully melted and the ingredients are combined, then pour it into a clean jar or tin. Once the salve has cooled and solidified, apply it to the affected area as needed.

So there you have it, some of the most common types of insect bites, and the best herbal remedies to help soothe and heal them. Of course, these remedies aren't a substitute for medical attention if you're experiencing a severe reaction or other symptoms. But for mild to moderate insect bites, they can be a great natural alternative to traditional over-the-counter treatments. So next time you get a mosquito bite or a tick bite, try reaching for one of these herbal remedies and see how it works for you.

leg cramps

LEG CRAMPS ARE a common problem experienced by many people, particularly athletes, seniors, and pregnant women. They are often characterized by sudden, intense pain in the leg muscles, making it difficult to move and function normally. But did you know that there are different types of leg cramps, and each may have its own causes and best herbal remedies?

The most common type of leg cramps is called idiopathic leg cramps. This means that the exact cause of the cramps is unknown. However, certain factors may contribute to their occurrence, such as dehydration, muscle fatigue, and electrolyte imbalances and if you're low on electrolytes like calcium, magnesium, and potassium. For these types of leg cramps, there are several herbal remedies that can help relieve symptoms and prevent future occurrences.

One of the most effective herbal remedies for idiopathic leg cramps is **Magnesium**. This mineral plays a vital role in muscle function and relaxation, and a deficiency can lead to cramping. You can increase your magnesium intake by consuming foods like leafy greens, nuts, seeds, and whole grains, or by taking a magnesium supplement.

Another great herbal remedy for leg cramps is **Ginger**. This root has anti-inflammatory properties and can help reduce pain and swelling associated with muscle cramps. Ginger can be consumed as a tea, added to smoothies or other beverages, or taken in supplement form.

For athletes or individuals who experience leg cramps due to intense physical activity, **Arnica** is a great herbal remedy. Arnica is a natural anti-inflammatory and pain reliever that can help reduce muscle soreness and inflammation. It can be applied topically as a cream or ointment, or taken in supplement form.

Another common type of leg cramp is nocturnal leg cramps. These cramps typically occur at night, often waking the sufferer from sleep. They may be caused by dehydration, overuse of leg muscles, or certain medications. For nocturnal leg cramps, there are several herbal remedies that can help alleviate symptoms and prevent future occurrences.

One of the best herbal remedies for nocturnal leg cramps is **Valerian** root. Valerian root has sedative properties and can help promote relaxation and restful sleep. It can be consumed as a tea or taken in supplement form.

Another great herbal remedy for nocturnal leg cramps is **Chamomile**. This herb has anti-inflammatory properties and can help reduce pain and swelling associated with muscle cramps. Chamomile can be consumed as a tea or taken in supplement form.

For pregnant women experiencing leg cramps, the cause may be related to changes in hormone levels and increased pressure on the legs.

One great herbal remedy for leg cramps during pregnancy is **Lavender** oil. It has soothing properties and can help promote relaxation and reduce muscle tension. It can be applied topically as a massage oil or added to a warm bath.

Another effective herbal remedy for leg cramps during pregnancy is **Black Cohosh**. With its anti-inflammatory properties it can help reduce pain and swelling associated with muscle cramps. It can be consumed as a tea or taken in supplement form.

One last method is simply a bar of soap! I know many people who swear by this. Place a bar of soap, and it can be almost any bar of soap, under your bed sheet or in a sock near your leg - and that's it! There is no scientific evidence to support this but I know many people who this seems to have helped.

Leg cramps can be a real pain. Whether you're experiencing idiopathic leg cramps, nocturnal leg cramps, or leg cramps during pregnancy. Try incorporating some of these remedies into your daily routine and see how they work for you!

thirty-seven
memory & focus

IMPROVING your memory and focus is something that herbal medicine excels at. You will notice how many scientifically-backed herbs are in this chapter compared to some others.

This may not be surprising to you. Many drugs and nootropics have plant origins. Caffeine is the most popular social drug in the world, and it has been proven to improve memory and focus.

It also has its roots in herbal medicine, with green and black tea being drunk in China and India and coffee used in South America. Cocaine, which despite all its obvious negatives, is incredibly effective at improving focus and memory and was used in herbal medicine for exactly that (though in a much less concentrated form).

This chapter has split the herbal remedies into two groups:

- Herbal remedies for memory
- Herbal remedies for focus/cognition

But several herbs in these lists will provide both benefits, though almost always one benefit is stronger than the other. Ginkgo Biloba has a significant effect on memory and only a slight effect on focus and cognition, so it is only listed in the memory section.

Herbs for Memory

Caffeine is rarely seen as a form of herbal medicine, yet black tea contains caffeine, as does green tea. Coffee might not feel like a herbal remedy, yet is it not just an infusion of a plant? Either way, caffeine is an effective natural remedy for improving certain aspects of memory.

Spatial memory is the form of memory required for remembering where you have left your car keys or how to get from your house to work. Caffeine appears to be very effective at improving this form of memory.

It is also effective at helping your perceptual memory. This is the form of memory you use to remember your favorite song or what your uncle's face looks like.

A very interesting study in 2010 found that drinking **Blueberry** juice had a pronounced effect on memory in older people [40]. Interestingly, the study also found that the participants reported higher subjective wellbeing scores afterward. Meaning that blueberry juice may also help with depression.

Ginger really is the spice that keeps on giving! 400 to 800mg of ginger extract taken daily was shown to be effective at improving memory in older women. While there are no studies as of yet, finding out if ginger teas or consuming ginger in food have similar results would be fascinating.

Another herb for older individuals, **Ginkgo Biloba** has quite a lot of evidence to support its ability to improve short-term memory. It can also help to improve your cognition (whatever age), so it could be a good supplement to take before an exam.

Bacopa Monnieri is a herbal supplement that can help people of all ages to improve their memory. It is very popular in nootropic communities and is also used in ayurvedic medicine. In India, bacopa monnieri is taken with ghee because it is fat-soluble.

Black Cumin or Nigella sativa is a spice that is often used to lower cholesterol and improve blood pressure. But it also appears to help improve memory and recall in older people.

Red Clover extract has shown some evidence of being able to improve memory, but more research is required. Adding 5 grams of the plant to boiled water and letting it brew is a good way to take it, and you may get some great results.

As always, check the law before considering whether to use this or not. But **Cannabis** may actually be an effective herb for improving memory.

There is a lot of confusion about cannabis. It is certainly true that if you take enough cannabis to become intoxicated, your short-term memory can be affected in the same way that your coordination can be affected when you drink too much.

But sensible use of cannabis over time appears to be beneficial for memory in the long term. More research is required to find out the ideal dosage and whether it works for everyone, but it's certainly something to keep an eye out for in the future.

The idea that eating chocolate can improve memory seems too good to be true. But there may be a connection between **Cocoa extract** and memory formation. Some studies have shown an improvement while others have failed to find a statistical difference, but cocoa extract has many other benefits, so at worst, you should still see health benefits.

Turning to a much less controversial herb, we have **Ashwagandha**. This herb is usually used to treat anxiety and to help with sleep. But it also appears to be effective in improving memory. Taking 300-500 mg of Ashwagandha root extract should help you to see some results.

Lemon balm (Melissa officinalis) is a herbal tea that may be of some use in improving memory. Several studies have shown that lemon balm tea can help to improve memory formation. 300mg is a typical dosage, or you can just follow the instructions if you are buying it from a store.

While there isn't much scientific evidence for it working, many herbalists recommend **Peppermint** oil for improving memory. Try it out for yourself; add a few drops to some water or a diffuser and see what happens.

Herbs for Cognition/Focus

Cognition is a psychological term for brain power (this is a simplified definition), and it is a bit of an umbrella term for a number of mental processes. It can involve problem-solving, reasoning, judging, paying attention, or focusing.

Scientific studies rarely look specifically at focus, but rather they look for whether a herb or plant can improve cognition. This is why this section of the chapter is titled cognition/focus.

Caffeine is, of course, one of the best cognitive enhancers out there, and in high doses, it can be very effective at improving focus. **Green tea catechins** are also known to be effective at improving focus and cognition.

Rhodiola Rosea works in a similar way to caffeine, banishing fatigue and allowing you to focus better. It is very effective if stress and anxiety have caused fatigue, either physical or mental. 280-680 mg of Rhodiola Rosea extract have been shown to be most effective.

A herb that is used a lot in Traditional Chinese Medicine is **Panax Ginseng** which is used to boost mood, banish fatigue, improve cognition, and it is also used for its ability to top up your immune system. 200-400mg taken in capsule form appear to be effective.

The next herb to look at is **Kava**, which plays an important role in Polynesian culture, and also appears to be an effective herb for anxiety. Studies have shown that kava may be helpful with improving focus in people whose mood has been affected by anxiety or depression.

Kava is consumed in a number of different ways depending on which island you are on, and the strength can vary, with fresh kava being considerably stronger than the kava found in herbal supplements.

Nigella Sativa, better known as **Black Cumin**, is a spice that is used a lot in herbal medicine. It has a minor effect on attention and on overall cognition. It can be taken as a seed extract or seed oil.

Kanna is a herb that is very popular in South Africa and has been used by hunter-gatherers in Africa for hundreds of years. It is usually chewed, but it works well as a tea or a tincture.

It is very effective at dealing with anxiety and helping you to focus during stressful situations.

thirty-eight
menopause

I OFTEN SAY that a topic needs so much more than a chapter and this topic is definitely one of those. We have peri-menopause, and 'post-menopause' and each is different, with many different possible effects from memory to hair loss and of course depression. In this chapter I will take a look at the menopause generally and cover the most common problems and conditions.

Menopause is something that all women go through, but not many of us like to talk about it. And who can blame us? The menopause can be uncomfortable and even downright painful at times. But don't worry. As a herbal author, I'm here to shed some light on the subject and give you some tips on how to manage your symptoms naturally.

First things first, let's talk about what menopause actually is. Menopause is a natural biological process that marks the end of menstruation and fertility in women. It typically occurs between the ages of 45 and 55, but can happen earlier or later. During menopause, a woman's body produces less estrogen and progesterone, which can cause a variety of symptoms.

So, what kind of symptoms are we talking about here? Well, they can vary from woman to woman, but some common ones include hot flashes, night sweats, mood swings, vaginal dryness, and difficulty sleeping. And let's not forget about the increased risk of osteoporosis and heart disease that comes with the hormonal changes of menopause.

But fear not. There are herbs that can help alleviate some of these uncomfortable symptoms. Let's take a look at some of the most common symptoms and the herbs that can help manage them.

Hot Flashes

The dreaded hot flash. It's a sudden feeling of warmth that spreads over the body, often accompanied by sweating and a rapid heartbeat. **Black Cohosh** has been used to manage the frequency and severity of hot flashes in menopausal women. You can take it in supplement form or drink it as a tea. **Chasteberry** and **Wild Yam** can all also help with hot flashes and mood changes, and can also be taken as a tea (Yam is used in some HRT therapies because it is used to make 17 beta-estradiol, which is body identical).

Night Sweats

Night sweats are like hot flashes, but they happen at night. They can be disruptive to sleep and leave you feeling tired and groggy in the morning. **Sage** can reduce the frequency and intensity of night sweats in menopausal women.

You can drink it as a tea or take it in supplement form. **Red Clover,** like Sage, can be taken as a tea dried to help with hot flashes and night sweats.

Mood Swings and depression

Mood swings can be a real rollercoaster ride during menopause. One moment you're feeling on top of the world, and the next you're in tears for no reason.

Red Clover extract would be a good herb to try if you are suffering from depression as a result of the menopause. Studies in menopausal women found that red clover extract was able to reduce depression by up to 80%. Two doses of 40mg of pure isoflavones are effective, or 5 grams of the whole plant.

St. John's Wort has also been shown to improve mood and reduce anxiety in menopausal women. You can take it in supplement form, but be sure to talk to your doctor first if you're on any medications.

Vaginal Dryness

Vaginal dryness is a common symptom of menopause and can make sex uncomfortable or even painful. A great herb that helps here is an oil - Evening Primrose Oil. It contains gamma-linolenic acid (GLA), which can help improve vaginal lubrication. You can take it in supplement form or apply it directly to the vagina as a cream.

Difficulty Sleeping

Sleep disturbances are another common symptom of menopause. Whether you're having trouble falling asleep or staying asleep, it can leave you feeling tired and irritable during the day. This time, you can try Valerian. This herb is known to improve sleep quality and reduce the time it takes to fall asleep in menopausal women. You can take it in supplement form or as a tea.

Menopause can cause a variety of changes in a woman's body beyond the common symptoms I mention above. For example:

Skin changes: As women age, their skin becomes thinner, drier, and less elastic. Menopause can exacerbate these changes due to falling estrogen and progesterone, leading to wrinkles, dryness, and age spots. One herb that may help improve skin health during menopause is **Gotu Kola**.

This herb can improve skin elasticity, hydration, and collagen production. A study published in the Journal of Medicinal Food found that taking Gotu Kola supplements for 12 weeks improved skin hydration and elasticity in middle-aged women. You can take Gotu Kola as a tea or as a supplement.

Hair changes: Menopause can cause changes in hair texture, thickness, and growth. Many women experience hair thinning or loss during this time. One herb that may help promote healthy hair growth is **Saw Palmetto**. This herb has been traditionally used to treat hair loss in men and women.

A study published in the Journal of Alternative and Complementary Medicine found that topical application of Saw Palmetto extract improved hair growth in men and women with androgenetic alopecia (hair loss). You can take Saw Palmetto in supplement form or apply it topically as an oil or cream.

Another remedy is **Rosemary**. Mix a few spoons of Rosemary with Apple Cider Vinegar and pat onto your head with a cotton bud, leave for 10 minutes, then wash your hair as normal. There is more on hair loss in that chapter.

Joint pain: Menopause can exacerbate joint pain and stiffness, particularly in women who have already experienced joint problems.

Turmeric, as we know contains curcumin, a powerful anti-inflammatory compound. A study published in the Journal of Medicinal Food found that taking a Turmeric supplement for 8 weeks reduced joint pain and inflammation in middle-aged women with knee osteoarthritis. You can take Turmeric in supplement form or use it as a spice in cooking.

Digestive issues: Menopause can also cause digestive problems, such as bloating, constipation, and diarrhea. A study published in the Journal of Gastroenterology found that taking **Peppermint oil** capsules for 4 weeks improved symptoms of irritable bowel syndrome (IBS), including bloating, abdominal pain, and gas. You can take Peppermint as a supplement or as a tea.

Memory and cognitive decline: Menopause can cause changes in cognitive function, including memory loss and difficulty concentrating.

One herb that may help improve cognitive function is **Ginkgo Biloba**. This herb has been traditionally used to enhance memory and cognitive function. A study published in the Journal of Psychopharmacology found that taking Ginkgo Biloba supplements for 6 weeks improved memory and cognitive function in middle-aged women. You can take Ginkgo Biloba in supplement form or drink it as a tea.

thirty-nine
menstruation

MENSTRUATION IS a natural process that occurs in the female body, where the lining of the uterus is shed and flows out of the body through the vagina. This usually happens once a month, and the duration and intensity can vary from woman to woman.

While menstruation is a completely normal and necessary part of reproductive health, it can also come with a variety of uncomfortable symptoms.

Let's dive a little deeper into the specific conditions that women can experience during menstruation, and the herbs that can help alleviate them.

Cramp

First up, let's talk about menstrual cramps. These are due to a number of things, including hormonal changes and inflammation. The good news is that there are several herbs that can help alleviate these cramps. One of the most well-known is **Cramp bark**. As the name suggests, this herb has a long history of use for menstrual cramps, as well as other types of cramps and spasms.

The bark of the Cramp bark plant contains several active compounds, including valerenic acid, which has muscle-relaxing properties. Cramp bark works by relaxing smooth muscle tissue, which can help alleviate the contractions that cause menstrual cramps. You can try taking a cramp bark supplement or drinking cramp bark tea.

Another favorite is the ever-present **Ginger**. Because it contains compounds that have anti-inflammatory effects, it can can help reduce the severity of menstrual cramps. You can enjoy ginger in tea, or try adding it to your meals during your period.

Heavy bleeding

Many women can experience heavy bleeding during menstruation which can be due to hormonal imbalances and certain medical conditions, also known as menorrhagia. Some of the most common causes include:

Fibroids are noncancerous growths that develop in or around the uterus. They can cause heavy bleeding, as well as pain and discomfort during menstruation.

Endometriosis is a condition in which the tissue that lines the uterus grows outside of it, often on the ovaries, fallopian tubes, or other organs in the pelvic area. It can cause heavy bleeding, as well as pain, cramping, and infertility.

Adenomyosis is when the tissue that lines the uterus grows into the muscular wall of the uterus. It can cause heavy bleeding, as well as pain and discomfort during menstruation.

Polyps are small growths that can develop on the lining of the uterus. They can cause heavy bleeding, as well as irregular periods and pain during menstruation.

Thyroid disorders, such as hypothyroidism or hyperthyroidism, can cause hormonal imbalances that can lead to heavy bleeding during menstruation.

If you are experiencing heavy bleeding during menstruation, it's important to determine the underlying cause. In some cases, treatment may include medication, hormonal therapy, or surgery. However, in many cases, natural remedies like herbs can also be helpful in alleviating symptoms and supporting overall menstrual health.

One herb that can help heavy bleeding is **Yarrow**. Yarrow contains compounds that have been shown to help reduce bleeding and promote healing. You can try drinking yarrow tea or taking a yarrow supplement.

Bloating, another common symptom, can be caused by water retention. Fennel contains compounds that can help reduce inflammation and promote digestion, which can help reduce bloating. You can try drinking Fennel tea or adding Fennel to your meals during your period.

Mood swings and fatigue

Mood swings are another common symptom of menstruation, and can be caused by hormonal fluctuations. One herb that can help support mood during this time is **Chamomile**. Chamomile contains compounds that have been shown to have a calming effect on the nervous system, which can help alleviate symptoms of anxiety and irritability. You can try drinking Chamomile tea or taking a chamomile supplement.

Finally, fatigue and low energy are common during menstruation, and can be caused by hormonal changes and blood loss.

One herb that can help support energy levels during this time is **Maca** root. Maca is a root vegetable that has been used for centuries to support energy and vitality.

During menstruation, many women experience fatigue as a result of hormonal changes and the body's increased energy demands. Maca can help alleviate this fatigue by supporting the adrenal glands, which are responsible for regulating the body's stress response and energy levels. By supporting the adrenal glands, Maca can help the body better adapt to the demands of menstruation and maintain energy levels throughout the day.

In addition to its fatigue-fighting properties, Maca is also thought to have several other health benefits, including improving mood, supporting fertility, and enhancing libido. It can be taken as a supplement, added to smoothies or other beverages, or used in cooking.

As with any herbal remedy, it's important to talk to your healthcare provider before adding Maca to your routine.

forty
motion sickness

TRAVEL SICKNESS, also known as motion sickness, is caused by a disagreement between the senses in your body that help you maintain balance and orientation. The inner ear, which helps regulate balance and spatial orientation, may sense motion from the movement of the vehicle you're traveling in, such as a car, boat, or plane. However, your eyes may not be able to see the movement or motion that your inner ear is sensing. It is this conflict between the senses that can motion sickness.

Symptoms of travel sickness can include nausea, vomiting, dizziness, sweating, and headache. These symptoms usually improve once the motion stops, but can be uncomfortable and disruptive in the meantime.

Children, pregnant women, and people with a history of migraines or inner ear problems are often more susceptible to this condition.

Other factors that can contribute to motion sickness, and increase its severity, include anxiety or stress related to travel, strong smells, and poor ventilation.

There are several strategies that can help prevent or alleviate the problem, such as focusing on the horizon or a fixed point in the distance, avoiding strong smells or spicy foods before and during travel, staying hydrated, and getting fresh air if possible.

There are also over-the-counter medications, but both **Ginger** and **Peppermint** are my favorites, especially Ginger. You can take Ginger supplements, chew on ginger candy or ginger chews, or drink ginger tea. You can also try sipping on ginger ale or ginger beer, but be sure to choose a brand that contains real ginger.

forty-one
nausea & vomiting

NAUSEA AND VOMITING are symptoms of illness or your brain's way of removing something that is bad from you. If you know why you are vomiting or feeling sick (for example, you drank too much last night or you just got off a rollercoaster), then some herbal remedies may make you feel better.

If you don't know why you are vomiting or feeling nauseated, then you may want to talk to a doctor first.

The most commonly used herbal remedy for nausea is **Ginger**. You can eat it or drink it as Ginger tea. It is great for preventing sea sickness too.

Adding a teaspoon of **Cloves** to boiling water can make clove tea, which is a well-known herbal remedy for nausea and vomiting. Let the tea brew for 10 minutes to get the correct strength.

The smell of **lemons** has been shown to reduce nausea. You can either use a fresh lemon or a lemon extract or essential oil.

Spices such as **Cinnamon** and **Cumin** are also used to treat nausea, but you may need quite a large dosages, which makes them impractical.

Fennel tea, where you add a teaspoon of fennel seeds to boiling water, may help to reduce nausea and prevent vomiting.

Peppermint and **Lavender** essential oils are another potential method for reducing nausea (you can also use Clove oil). Place the oils in a diffuser and lie down to get the best results. You can also make Peppermint tea using a teaspoon of Peppermint and some boiled water.

Nausea is one area where acupuncture may be of use. Obviously, it requires some forethought, but if you know that you are going to be nauseated (morning sickness, for example), you can book an appointment for the next day.

One plant that may prove helpful depending on the laws in your country is **Cannabis**. A 2020 study on patients who were undergoing chemotherapy found that a mixture of CBD and THC extract helped to reduce nausea and vomiting. The only downsides were dizziness and sleepiness afterward.

forty-two
pain relief

PAIN IS one of the most common health problems people seek medication and herbal remedies for. This is because pain is a natural response of the body to an injury or a disease, and it's essential for our survival. It tells us that something is wrong and that we need to take action to fix it. Many of the conditions detailed in this book address some of the specific problems but here is a general overview of pain.

Pain can be acute, which means that it is sudden and severe, or chronic, which means that it lasts for a long time, usually more than three months. The causes of pain can vary, and the way the body responds to it can also differ. For example, the pain you feel when you stub your toe is different from the pain you feel when you have a headache.

Acute pain is usually caused by an injury, such as a cut, burn, or broken bone. When you injure yourself, the body releases chemicals called prostaglandins that cause inflammation and pain. This is why your injured area may become red, swollen, and painful. The pain is your body's way of telling you to protect the injured area and to give it time to heal.

Chronic pain, on the other hand, can be caused by many different conditions, such as arthritis, fibromyalgia, and neuropathy. In some cases, there may not be an identifiable cause, but the pain is still real and can be debilitating. Chronic pain can also cause other problems, such as anxiety, depression, and sleep disturbances, which can further impact a person's quality of life.

When it comes to treating pain, there are many options available. As a herbalist, I believe that natural remedies can be very effective in relieving pain without the side effects that can come with prescription or over-the-counter drugs. Here are some herbal remedies that have proven science to help with pain:

As we know by now, Turmeric contains an active ingredient called curcumin, which has anti-inflammatory properties. Inflammation is a major cause of pain, so taking turmeric supplements or adding turmeric to your diet can help relieve pain caused by inflammation. You can also make a turmeric tea by boiling a teaspoon of turmeric powder in a cup of water for 10 minutes.

Ginger, another familiar herb, has anti-inflammatory properties. It contains compounds called gingerols and shogaols, which can help reduce pain and inflammation. You can take ginger supplements or drink ginger tea by boiling sliced ginger in water for 10 minutes.

White willow bark contains a natural compound called salicin, which is similar to aspirin. Salicin can help relieve pain and reduce inflammation. You can take white willow bark supplements or make a tea by boiling a teaspoon of white willow bark in a cup of water for 10 minutes.

Capsaicin is the compound that gives chili peppers their spicy kick. It can help relieve pain by blocking the transmission of pain signals from the nerves to the brain. You can find capsaicin creams and ointments at health food stores or online.

Lavender, another familiar herb by now, has long been used as a natural remedy for pain and stress. It contains compounds that have a calming effect on the body and can help reduce pain and inflammation. You can use lavender essential oil by adding a few drops to a carrier oil, such as coconut or jojoba oil, and massaging it into the affected area.

forty-three
sinusitis

SINUSITIS IS a common condition that causes inflammation of the sinuses, which are the air-filled spaces in the skull that are connected to the nasal passages.

Sinuses are lined with cilia, tiny hair-like structures that help move mucus out of the sinuses and into the nasal passages. When the sinuses become inflamed, the cilia can become damaged, leading to a buildup of mucus and a greater risk of infection.

This inflammation can cause a range of unpleasant symptoms, such as nasal congestion, headaches, facial pain, and a fever.

The most common causes of sinusitis are viral infections, allergies, and bacterial infections. Let's take a closer look at each of these causes and explore the best herbal remedies for each.

Viral infections

Viral infections are the most common cause of sinusitis. These infections are caused by viruses that infect the respiratory tract, and they can lead to inflammation and congestion of the sinuses. The symptoms of viral sinusitis usually clear up on their own within a week or two.

The best herbs for treating viral sinusitis are those with antiviral properties. Some of the most effective herbs include **Echinacea**, **Elderberry**, and **Licorice** root. Echinacea can help boost the immune system and fight off viruses, while Elderberry has been shown to inhibit the replication of viruses. Licorice root has antiviral and anti-inflammatory properties and can help reduce inflammation in the sinuses.

Recipe

To prepare a tea with these herbs, combine one teaspoon of dried Echinacea, Elderberry, and Licorice root in a cup of boiling water. Steep for 10 minutes, strain, and drink up to three cups a day.

Source: The Journal of Alternative and Complementary Medicine

Allergies

Allergies are another common cause of sinusitis. Allergens such as pollen, dust, and animal dander can trigger an allergic reaction, leading to inflammation and congestion of the sinuses. The symptoms of allergic sinusitis can be similar to those of viral sinusitis, but they tend to be more persistent.

The best herbs for treating allergic sinusitis are those with antihistamine and anti-inflammatory properties and some of the most effective herbs include stinging **Nettle**, **Butterbur**, and **Eyebright**.

Stinging Nettle has been shown to reduce inflammation and inhibit histamine release, while Butterbur can help reduce nasal congestion and improve breathing. Eyebright is a natural antihistamine that can help reduce inflammation and relieve sinus pressure.

<u>Recipe</u>

To prepare a tea with these herbs, combine one teaspoon of dried stinging nettle, butterbur, and eyebright in a cup of boiling water. Steep for 10 minutes, strain, and drink up to three cups a day.

Bacterial Infections

Bacterial infections are less common than viral or allergic sinusitis, but they can be more serious. Bacterial infections can cause a buildup of pus in the sinuses, leading to more severe symptoms such as fever, facial pain, and a persistent cough. Antibiotics are usually prescribed to treat bacterial sinusitis.

Herbs can help support the immune system and promote healing. Some of the best herbs for bacterial sinusitis include **Goldenseal, Garlic,** and **Thyme**. Goldenseal has antibacterial properties and can help reduce inflammation in the sinuses. Garlic has been shown to have antibacterial and antiviral properties, while thyme can help clear mucus from the respiratory tract and support respiratory health.

<u>Recipe</u>

To prepare a tea with these herbs, combine one teaspoon of dried goldenseal, garlic, and thyme in a cup of boiling water. Steep for 10 minutes, strain, and drink up to three cups a day.

Please note that these herbs are intended to support the immune system and promote healing, but they may not a substitute for medications prescribed by a healthcare provider.

Children

Sinuses are not fully developed at birth and continue to grow and develop until around age 20. This means that children are more susceptible to sinus infections due to their still-developing sinuses.

- **Chamomile** is a gentle herb that can help calm inflammation and soothe sinus discomfort. It also has antimicrobial properties that can help fight infections. Chamomile is safe for children of all ages and can be prepared as a tea or added to a warm compress.
- **Echinacea** is a popular herb for immune support and can be helpful in fighting off infections that can cause sinusitis. It is safe for children over the age of one and can be prepared as a tea or taken in a tincture form.
- **Elderberry** is another immune-boosting herb that can help fight off infections. It is safe for children over the age of one and can be prepared as a syrup or added to a warm compress.
- **Licorice root** is a soothing herb that can help calm inflammation and promote healing. It is safe for children over the age of six and can be prepared as a tea or added to a warm compress.

It is important to note that while these herbs are generally considered safe for children, it is always best to consult with a healthcare provider before giving any herbs to children, particularly if they have a pre-existing medical condition or are taking medication. Additionally, it is important to source herbs from a reputable supplier and to follow recommended dosages.

forty-four
skin conditions

YOUR SKIN IS AN INCREDIBLY important part of your integumentary system and is the body's largest organ. It has many functions, but these can be boiled down to the following:

- Regulates body temperature – sweating when you are hot, goosebumps when you are cold
- Sensation – pain, temperature, pressure, etc
- Immunity and protection – it keeps bad things out
- Allows movement

Skincare is often denigrated as vanity, but the truth is that protecting your skin is a vital aspect of health - protecting it from damage can make you feel more confident and happier.

Herbal medicine for the skin has been around for thousands of years. Ancient Egyptians used oil extracts to protect their skin from wrinkles 6,000 years ago!

When you look at Traditional Chinese Medicine, Ayurveda, and Native American Medicine, they all have specific herbs to treat the symptoms, but they also have theories as to what causes skin complaints in the first place.

Dry skin is a common skin condition that affects many people. The skin becomes dry when it loses its natural oils and moisture, resulting in flakiness, itching, and cracking. There are several causes of dry skin, including environmental factors, genetics, and underlying medical conditions.

This rest of this chapter will look at some herbal remedies for the following:

- Dry Skin
- Acne
- Pruritus (Itchy Skin)
- Eczema
- Psoriasis

But first, because I tend towards TCM when it comes to skin health and, according to TCM, your qi (vital energy) and blood must flow freely throughout the body and its organs to maintain the balance of yin (cooling) and yang (heating) elements.

This means that bad skin can be the result of an imbalance in the body's functions and bad skin can be caused by a number of different types of imbalances.

For example, if your body is failing to eliminate waste properly because of poor circulation of blood (qi) then your body will get rid of the toxins through your skin causing acne.

Or your body could be storing excess heat causing skin irritation. In this case, TCM advises that this is caused by your lungs because your lungs provide your skin with blood and qi. If the problem is caused by excess heat your are likely to see other inflammation in your body such as rashes. To reduce the heat you would eat 'yin', or cooling foods like cucumbers, celery, pears or lentils. These are moisture rich and help to cool your system. Avoid heating foods like caffeine, dairy and spicy foods.

Eczema and acne can be caused by "damp heat". You would eat Asparagus or Turnip and avoid cooling foods.

For a healthy skin you would use **Wolfberries** that are full of antioxidants and reduce the signs of aging. Or you could try **Mung beans**, another cooling legume that detoxifies your body and removes heat.

Another great plant to try is **Dandelion** and dandelion tea can be used instead of coffee. It has both detoxifying and diuretic properties that flushes out the kidney, liver and bladder and can reduce acne.

Dry Skin

As we age, our skin produces less oil, leading to dryness and fine lines. Hormonal imbalances, such as those that occur during pregnancy or menopause, can also cause dry skin.

These hormonal imbalances can lead to decreased oil production in the skin, leading to dryness and fine lines.

Evening primrose oil can help to alleviate the symptoms of dry skin caused by hormonal changes. It contains gamma-linolenic acid, an omega-6 fatty acid that can help to support the skin's natural moisture barrier. Evening primrose oil can be applied topically in the form of a cream or oil. It is should not be used by individuals with epilepsy or those who are taking blood-thinning medication.

Flaxseed oil contains omega-3 fatty acids that can help to support the skin's natural moisture barrier and reduce inflammation. Flaxseed oil can be applied topically in the form of a ream or oil, or taken orally as a supplement. It is generally considered safe for most people, but it may interact with certain medications, including blood-thinning medication.

Red clover contains compounds that can help to balance hormones and is often used during the menopause. Take it orally as a supplement or apply topically in the form of a cream or oil. However, it may interact with certain medications, including blood-thinning medication.

Environment can play a part too. Cold, dry air in the winter can strip the skin of its natural oils, causing it to become dry and itchy. Hot, dry air in the summer can also dehydrate the skin, leading to dryness and flakiness.

In this case try **Calendula, Chamomile or Comfrey.** Both Calendula and Chamomile can be applied topically in the form of a cream, oil, or tea and both may cause an allergic reaction in individuals with a sensitivity to plants in the Asteraceae family.

Comfrey can promote cell regeneration and soothe the skin, reducing inflammation and redness. Apply topically in the form of a cream or oil. However, it should be used with caution as it can be toxic when ingested or applied to broken skin.

Acne

Acne is a common skin condition that affects millions of people. It is characterized by the appearance of pimples, blackheads, and whiteheads on the face, neck, back, and chest. Acne is caused by a complex interplay of factors, including hormonal changes, genetics, bacteria, and lifestyle habits.

Hormonal changes play a crucial role in the development of acne. During puberty, androgen hormone levels increase, leading to the production of more oil (sebum) by the sebaceous glands. This can clog the pores and create an ideal environment for the growth of the bacteria Propionibacterium acnes, which can trigger inflammation and result in acne breakouts.

Genetics can also play a role in acne susceptibility, as the condition tends to run in families. Certain genetic variations may affect the way the body responds to hormonal changes and how susceptible the skin is to developing acne.

Lifestyle factors, such as diet, stress, and skin care habits, can also contribute to breakouts while a diet high in sugar and processed foods can trigger inflammation and exacerbate symptoms.

Stress can also be a trigger by causing hormonal imbalances and increasing sebum production and using products that are too harsh or not appropriate for your skin type can irritate the skin and trigger a breakout.

Herbs have been used for centuries to treat acne and its symptoms. Some of the most commonly used herbs for acne include:

- **Tea tree oil** has antimicrobial and anti-inflammatory properties and is most often used topically to treat pimples and other acne-related skin problems.
- **Green tea** contains antioxidants and anti-inflammatory compounds that can help reduce the redness and swelling associated with acne. It can be applied topically to the skin or consumed as a tea (see below).
- **Aloe vera** has anti-inflammatory and moisturizing properties. Apply topically to help soothe and hydrate the skin.
- **Witch hazel** is an astringent that helps to tighten and tone the skin. Applied topically to the skin it helps to reduce inflammation.
- **Turmeric** contains anti-inflammatory compounds that can help reduce the redness and swelling associated with acne. It

can be applied topically to the skin or consumed as a supplement to help soothe acne-prone skin.

Other teas include **Dandelion** - its diuretic properties and may help to flush toxins from the body - and **Lemon Balm** with antiviral and antibacterial properties which may help to reduce inflammation.

One of the best teas (which is technically not a herbal tea) that has been proven to help with acne caused by puberty is **Green Tea**. It is rich in antioxidants and anti-inflammatory compounds, such as epicatechin, gallate, and catechins, which have been shown to help reduce the redness and swelling associated with acne. In a study published in the Journal of Drugs in Dermatology, green tea was found to be effective in reducing the number of pimples and improving overall skin clarity in individuals with acne-prone skin

Another study published in the International Journal of Dermatology found that topical application of green tea extract reduced the number of pimples and improved skin texture in patients with moderate to severe acne.

In addition to its anti-inflammatory properties, green tea has antimicrobial effects that help to fight the bacteria Propionibacterium acnes, which is a major contributor to acne breakouts. Drinking green tea or applying it topically to the skin can help soothe acne-prone skin and reduce the appearance of pimples.

However, it is important to note that green tea is not appropriate for everyone and may not be safe for individuals with certain medical conditions. For example, green tea can interact with blood thinners and can increase the risk of bleeding in individuals taking these medications. Additionally, green tea may cause skin irritation in some individuals, particularly those with sensitive skin.

Pruritus (Itchy Skin)

Itchy skin can be an absolute nightmare to live with, particularly when you realize that your natural desire to scratch that itch will likely worsen things in the long term. There are numerous causes for pruritus. It is important to note that herbal medicine can only treat some of them.

Pruritus can sometimes be a symptom of an undiagnosed disease such as diabetes, lymphoma, liver disease, or anemia. It may also be the result of a psychiatric condition such as OCD or anxiety. Or it could be caused by an allergy. Nerve disorders such as multiple sclerosis can also cause pruritus .

But the most common causes of itchy skin are pretty mundane. Insect bites, hives, dry skin, or scars. Eczema and psoriasis are also causes, but they have their own sections.

If your arm (or whatever) has started to itch and you are fairly sure it's a minor issue, then using herbal remedies is a good idea. If the condition lasts a while, you may want to see your doctor to establish the cause.

There are three methods that you can use to treat itchy skin without using pharmaceuticals.

1. Treat the inflammation with herbal remedies
2. Cool the skin with poultices
3. Use herbs to relax and reduce stress or anxiety

Four herbal remedies that you can use to treat inflammation would be:

- **Colloidal Oatmeal** – Not exactly a herb, but colloidal oatmeal is a natural product derived from a plant! Colloidal oatmeal has been shown to reduce inflammation, and studies have shown that it can prevent itching and scaling [30]. You can add it to bathwater or apply it as a poultice.

- **Menthol** – Another anti-inflammatory, this can be applied topically or in a poultice.
- **Juniper Berries & Cloves** – A Native American remedy for itchy skin, these can be made into a salve (after performing oil extraction), or you could use a tincture on your skin.
- **Witch Hazel** - another Native American remedy, witch hazel can be used to sooth itchy skin but there is limited evidence that it can help specifically with eczema. This can be applied as an ointment, as the water distilled with the dried leaves, bark and twigs (Hamamelis water). There is evidence that applying a specific witch hazel ointment (Hametum) to the skin appears to improve symptoms of skin injury or irritated skin as effectively as a dexpanthenol ointment in children.

Using herbs to relax is only effective if your itchy skin is caused by anxiety, stress, or depression. Or if these issues are affecting your nutrition or sleep patterns.

Using essential oils such as **Lavender** to help you fall asleep could help your skin in the long term. **Valerian root** is a good herbal remedy for anxiety, as is **Chamomile**. Incidentally, you can apply chamomile topically to the skin to help with the itch.

Eczema

A cream prepared with **witch hazel** and phosphatidylcholine has been reported to be as effective as 1% hydrocortisone in the topical management of eczema, according to one double-blind trial however eczema is an umbrella term for a number of different skin conditions, each with a different cause. You have:

- Atopic dermatitis
- Contact dermatitis
- Neurodermatitis

And several more, but the first three are useful for this section. Contact dermatitis is caused by allergens, and it is best treated through avoidance of that allergen. If that allergen comes from soap or a detergent, swapping to a herbal salve may be beneficial.

Neurodermatitis has no known cause, but one theory is that it results from scratching the itch, making things worse. Using the herbal remedies we looked at in the pruritus section could help, as could the lifestyle changes (avoiding stress, sleeping better, reducing anxiety).

Atopic dermatitis is caused by a combination of dry skin and genetics; it can be exacerbated by scratching and bad health. As with neurodermatitis, using herbal remedies for pruritus can make a huge difference.

Atopic dermatitis can also be caused by hormonal changes, food allergies, and environmental factors. Consulting with a dermatologist or food allergen specialist should be your first step.

Psoriasis

Psoriasis is an auto-immune disease where your immune system begins to attack itself. The specific cause is unknown in this instance. It can cause red scaly patches on the skin, very dry areas of skin, a lot of itchiness and soreness, and even stiff joints.

Stress, bad sleep, illness, smoking, and injuries (such as sunburn or bug bites) can exacerbate problems or trigger them to come back. Psoriasis has no cure, but it can be managed.

Essential oils have been shown to reduce anxiety, which can help with/alongside pharmaceutical treatment. Regular sunshine can also help.

Oregon grape can be applied topically to the area to reduce the severity, as can **Aloe Vera** extract. **Epsom salts** in your bath are also effective for reducing inflammation.

Taking **Turmeric** capsules or brewing turmeric tea can help with inflammation during a flare-up.

Other teas to consider include **Burdock, Calendula, Licorice root** which are all also used to help with psoriasis. They have anti-inflammatory properties that can help to reduce skin irritation. **Oat straw** can also help to moisturize the skin.

Finally, for skin problems Here are a few herbal tea recipes that may help with dry skin:

1. Lavender is an herb that is used to help with relaxation and to improve sleep. It has also been used to help with dry skin. To make lavender tea, steep 1-2 teaspoons of dried lavender flowers in 8 ounces of hot water for 5-10 minutes.
2. Nettle tea, known to help with allergies and to support overall health, can also help with dry skin. To make the tea, steep 1-2 teaspoons of dried nettle leaves in 8 ounces of hot water for 5-10 minutes.
3. Almond milk is a natural moisturizer that has been traditionally used to help with dry skin. To make almond milk tea, combine 1 cup of unsweetened almond milk, 1 cup of water, and 1-2 teaspoons of your favorite tea leaves in a saucepan. Bring to a boil, then reduce the heat and let it simmer for 5-10 minutes. Strain the tea and enjoy.

forty-five
sleep & insomnia

INSOMNIA IS DEFINED as a sustained period of poor sleep. It can involve waking up multiple times during the night, struggling to fall asleep, feeling more tired than usual after waking up (a sign that you are waking up multiple times without realizing it) and feeling tired and irritable during the day.

There are many causes of insomnia. Noise issues, an uncomfortable bed, uncomfortable temperatures in your room, drug use (alcohol and caffeine included), or disrupted sleep schedules resulting from shift work or jet lag.

The biggest cause of insomnia though is stress, anxiety, or depression. These causes are particularly difficult as not only are they harder to deal with, but insomnia can actually make them worse, creating a vicious cycle.

There are many different treatments for insomnia, and it is important that you attempt to fix some of the simpler ones first, as this may cure your insomnia quickly.

Examples of this include:

- Purchasing a more comfortable bed and pillows
- Regulating the temperature in your room
- Reducing noise (including turning off loud electrical items)
- Create a sleep routine – having a bedtime can actually help you fall asleep quicker as your body will get used to falling asleep at the same time.
- Avoid caffeine or any stimulants for 6-8 hours before bedtime
- Avoiding overeating before bed – digestion of food can make sleeping harder
- Avoid overconsumption of alcohol – it too can make sleep difficult, particularly if you are drinking late at night.
- Meditation – There is lots of evidence that guided breathing exercises before bedtime can help you to fall asleep quicker

If you have tried all of this and you are still struggling, then the cause of your insomnia may be the result of stress, anxiety, or depression. If you do shift work, then it may not be caused by stress, anxiety, or depression, but the following herbal remedies may help anyway.

When we're feeling stressed or anxious, our bodies produce more cortisol, a hormone that can keep us awake and alert. This can make it difficult to fall asleep or stay asleep, even if we're tired. In this case, herbal remedies that can help reduce stress and promote relaxation may be helpful. For example, **Chamomile** tea has been shown to have a calming effect on the body and may help promote sleep and, **Passionflower** and **Valerian** root are often used to help calm the mind and promote relaxation.

Another common cause of sleep problems is pain. If you're experiencing chronic pain, it can be difficult to get comfortable enough to fall asleep, or you may wake up in the middle of the night in pain. In this case, herbs that can help alleviate pain may be helpful. For example, **Turmeric** has anti-inflammatory properties and may help reduce pain and inflammation in the body. Similarly, **Ginger** has been shown to have pain-relieving properties and may be helpful for those experiencing pain-related sleep problems.

Sleep apnea is a sleep disorder characterized by pauses in breathing during sleep, often caused by a blocked airway. This can lead to snoring, gasping, or choking during sleep, which can disrupt the sleep cycle and lead to daytime sleepiness or fatigue. In this case, herbs that can help improve respiratory function may be helpful. For example, **Eucalyptus** has been shown to have a bronchodilating effect, which can help open up the airways and improve breathing. Similarly, **Peppermint** may help reduce inflammation in the airways and improve breathing function.

Restless leg syndrome is a sleep disorder characterized by an irresistible urge to move the legs, often accompanied by discomfort or a tingling sensation. This can make it difficult to fall asleep or stay asleep, and can lead to daytime sleepiness or fatigue. In this case, herbs that can help promote relaxation and reduce the sensation of discomfort may be helpful. For example, **Magnesium** has been shown to help relax muscles and may be helpful for those experiencing restless leg syndrome. Similarly, and again, **Passionflower** and **Valerian** root may help promote relaxation and reduce discomfort.

Another common cure for insomnia is melatonin, a peptide hormone and neurotransmitter produced in the body. Low melatonin levels can lead to insomnia, so supplementation with melatonin may help address this.

You could, of course, just purchase a melatonin supplement, or you could alter your diet to eat more foods that contain melatonin, such as tomatoes, cereal, olive oil, and cherries. Beer and wine are also good sources of melatonin, but they can also disrupt sleep so they are not the best option.

Herbal supplements that can increase melatonin include **Shiya tea leaf**, and **Panax Notoginseng**. Both are supplements used in Traditional Chinese Medicine to reduce anxiety and improve sleep.

Shiya tea leaf can be drunk as regular tea, and it tastes great. 3-5g of tea leaves added to 125ml of boiling water will help with insomnia and is a great pre-bedtime drink.

Panax notoginseng can be mixed with water, or it can be taken in pill form; 1-3g is a standard dosage.

Valarian Root brewed into a tea or taken as a capsule is a very common herbal remedy for insomnia, with good results in women but less so in men. Take 450mg one hour before bed.

Other herbal remedies you may want to try include **Chaste Berry**, **Lavender**, and **Ashwagandha**.

forty-six
sore throat

THERE ARE many reasons that you might find yourself with sore throat. The most common ones are covered in this chapter along with the best herbs to consider.

Viral infection

A viral infection can cause inflammation in the throat, leading to soreness, pain, and difficulty swallowing.

When a viral infection, such as the common cold or the flu, enters the body, it triggers an immune response. The body's immune system recognizes the virus as foreign and begins to produce antibodies to fight off the infection.

This immune response can cause inflammation in the throat, which can lead to soreness, pain, and difficulty swallowing and it can cause other symptoms such as congestion, runny nose, and coughing. These symptoms can also irritate the throat and exacerbate the soreness and pain.

Elderberry has been shown to be effective for reducing the severity and duration of viral infections, including those that cause a sore throat. Its active ingredients include flavonoids and anthocyanins and it high in antioxidants. The flavonoids in elderberry have been shown to stimulate the production of cytokines such as interferons and inter-leukins, which play an important role in the body's immune response to viral infections - they help regulate the immune response.

Interestingly, as well as triggering the production of beneficial cytokines that help fight off viral infections, it also reduces the production of inflammatory cytokines that can contribute to inflammation and related symptoms.

Inflammatory cytokines are proteins that can trigger inflammation and it is this which can contribute to sore throat and other symptoms of viral infections.

It is therefore by both reducing the production of inflammatory cytokines, and increasing the production of the 'good' cytokines which boosts the immune response.

Elderberry can be taken in several forms, including as a syrup, capsule, or tea. Elderberry syrup is the most common form, and it can be found at many health food stores or made at home using fresh or dried elder-berries. Although Elderberry capsules and tea are also available, the syrup is the most effective form because it is more concentrated.

In general, the recommended dosage for elderberry syrup is one teaspoon for children and one tablespoon for adults, taken three to four times a day. Elderberry capsules are typically taken in doses of 500-1000 mg per day, while elderberry tea can be consumed two to three times a day. However, the dosage can vary depending on the the severity of symptoms.

Bacterial infection

Bacterial infections, such as strep throat, can require medical treatment, but certain herbs can also help with the symptoms. Like a viral infection the cause of the pain and discomfort it the result of the inflammatory response caused by the immune system.

Generally, a great herb for bacterial infections is **Echinacea**. It contains compounds called alkylamides and polysaccharides, which have been shown to reduce inflammation by stimulating the immune system.

It's important to note that Echinacea may interact with certain medications and should not be used if you have an autoimmune disease.

All of the following herbs can be taken as a tea, tincture or as a gargle.

- Echinacea - Strep Throat, Pharyngitis
- Ginger - Pharyngitis
- Goldenseal - Tonsilitis
- Licorice root - Strep Throat, Laryngitis
- Marshmallow root - Tonsilitis, Laryngitis, Dry throat
- Mullein - Tonsilitis
- Sage - Strep Throat, Laryngitis
- Slippery Elm - Tonsilitis , Laryngitis
- Thyme - Strep throat, Pharyngitis

Other herbs with an anti-inflammatory effect include Chamomile, Peppermint.

Strep Throat

This is one of the most common bacterial infections of the throat and it is caused by the bacteria Streptococcus pyogenes, which is also known as group A streptococcus.

Strep throat is characterized by a sudden onset of a sore throat, pain while swallowing, fever, and swollen lymph nodes in the neck.

If left untreated, strep throat can lead to complications such as rheumatic fever, kidney damage, and abscesses.

Echinacea is a great choice if you have strep throat and, with its immune-boosting properties, it can help the body fight off the infection.

Tonsilitis

This condition is characterized by inflammation and swelling of the tonsils, which are located at the back of the throat. It can be caused by several types of bacteria, including Streptococcus pyogenes, Staphylococcus aureus, and Haemophilus influenzae.

When the tonsils become infected, the body responds with an inflammatory response, causing the tonsils to become red, swollen, and painful. Other symptoms of tonsillitis may include fever, difficulty swallowing, and swollen lymph nodes in the neck.

One of the most effective herbs for Tonsilitis is **Goldenseal**. It's antimicrobial properties can help to fight off the bacteria causing the infection.

Don't overuse Goldenseal or take over a long period of time (take more than 3 times a day as a tea for more than two weeks).

Pharyngitis

As the name suggests, this is a bacterial infection that affects the pharynx, which is the part of the throat that connects the mouth and the nasal passages. It can be caused by several types of bacteria, including Streptococcus pyogenes, Corynebacterium diphtheriae, and

Mycoplasma pneumoniae and it is characterized by a sore throat, fever, and swollen lymph nodes in the neck.

When the pharynx becomes infected, the immune system response means that the pharynx become sred, swollen, and painful. Other symptoms of pharyngitis may include difficulty swallowing, hoarseness, and a cough.

Several herbs can be used to treat pharyngitis and one of the best is **Licorice root**, which has anti-inflammatory and antimicrobial properties.

As with all herbs, the appropriate dosage of licorice root can vary depending on several factors, including the form of the herb, the reason for use, and the individual's age and health status.

As a general guideline, a typical dosage of licorice root tea is 1-2 teaspoons of dried root per cup of water, steeped for 10-15 minutes. This can be consumed up to three times per day. However, it is important to note that the sweet taste of licorice can be quite strong, so some people may prefer to use it in capsule or tincture form instead.

It is generally recommended to use licorice root for short-term periods only, typically for up to four to six weeks at a time. This is because long-term or excessive use of licorice root can lead to side effects such as high blood pressure, low potassium levels, and an increased risk of heart disease.

Laryngitis

Laryngitis affects the larynx, which is the part of the throat that contains the vocal cords. It can be caused by several types of bacteria, including Streptococcus pyogenes and Haemophilus influenzae. Laryngitis is characterized by a hoarse or raspy voice, a cough, and a sore throat.

When the larynx becomes infected, the immune system response results in the larynx to become red, swollen, and painful. Other symptoms may include difficulty speaking, difficulty swallowing, and a fever.

As always, there are several herbs help. One of the most effective is marshmallow root with its soothing and anti-inflammatory properties.

As a general guideline, a safe dosage of **Marshmallow root** as a tea is around 1-2 teaspoons of dried root per cup of water. You can make the tea by steeping the marshmallow root in hot water for 10-15 minutes and then straining out the herb.

It is generally recommended to consume marshmallow root tea up to three times per day, depending on the severity of your symptoms. There is no consensus on the optimal duration of marshmallow root use, as this can vary depending on the person's condition and response to treatment. However, it is generally use marshmallow root for a limited period of time, such as several weeks, and then take a break to evaluate the effectiveness and any potential side effects.

Marshmallow root can also cause gastrointestinal side effects (amongst other things - see the chapter on Precautions) such as nausea, diarrhea, or stomach upset in some people. It means that you should start with a low dose and gradually increase it over time to minimize the risk of gastrointestinal side effects.

Allergies

Allergies, such as hay fever, can cause a sore throat due to postnasal drip. **Nettle** is a great herb for allergies as it has antihistamine and anti-inflammatory properties and it helps reduce inflammation and alleviate allergy symptoms. It contains compounds called histamine-releasing factors and lectins, which have been shown to reduce the amount of histamine produced by the body. It is histamine that causes allergy symptoms such as a runny nose, itchy eyes, and a sore throat.

You can find nettle in many forms such as tea or capsules.

Dry air

Believe it or not but dry air can cause a sore throat, especially during the winter months when indoor heating is used.

Marshmallow root should be your herb of choice if you suffer from a dry throat. It contains a high level of mucilage, a thick, gluey substance that can help reduce inflammation and promote healing. It's demulcent properties, which coat and soothe the throat, are great for a dry, scratchy throat.

You can take it as either a tea or a capsule.

Ulcers

Sometimes a sore throat can be caused by an ulcer, often due to a bacterial infection but it can also be the result of stress. A great herb for mouth ulcers is **sage**. I use this as a tea and swirl it around my mouth a few times. When you do this, don't swallow the tea - if it has captured the bacteria then expel the liquid, much as you would if you were using coconut oil as an oral cleanser. If I don't swirl it around my mouth then I simply drink it as a tea.

forty-seven
stomach ache

STOMACH PAIN and an upset stomach are two different conditions, although they are often used interchangeably to describe gastrointestinal discomfort.

While stomach pain and an upset stomach may share some symptoms, they are distinct conditions that require different treatments. For instance, an upset stomach may be treated with antacids or anti-nausea herbs, while stomach pain may require different herbal remedies or other treatments, depending on the underlying cause.

Stomach pain is a broad term used to describe discomfort or pain felt in the abdominal region. It can have various causes, including indigestion, acid reflux, stomach ulcers, inflammatory bowel disease, and many others. Stomach pain can be a sharp, cramp-like pain, a dull ache, or a burning sensation. Many of these are covered within the other chapters including the Gut, IBS, Acid Reflux, Constipation and Diarrhea

An upset stomach, on the other hand, is a more general term used to describe a range of symptoms related to gastrointestinal discomfort or pain in the upper abdomen. The discomfort is often described as a burning sensation or a feeling of fullness in the stomach and, often the result of indigestion, it can include symptoms such as nausea, vomiting, bloating, gas, and diarrhea.

Stomach pain

Stomach ulcers

Stomach ulcers are the result of a sore or hole in the lining of your stomach or small intestine and the most common cause is an infection with a bacteria called Helicobacter pylori. The symptoms of stomach ulcers include burning pain in the stomach, bloating, nausea, and vomiting.

There are several herbs that have been studied for their potential to help with stomach ulcers and one of the least well know is actually a vegetable. **Cabbage juice** has been found to have anti-inflammatory and anti-ulcer properties that may help reduce the size and severity of stomach ulcers. You can drink fresh cabbage juice or take cabbage juice supplements.

Other herbs that are known to help include **Licorice** root which has also been shown to help reduce the size and severity of stomach ulcers, as well as reduce the amount of stomach acid produced. Don't forget that long-term use of Licorice root can have side effects, such as high blood pressure and low potassium levels, so it's best to use it under the guidance of a healthcare professional.

Slippery Elm can help coat the lining of the stomach and protect it from further damage and **Chamomile** may help reduce inflammation and discomfort associated with stomach ulcers. All can be taken as a tea or capsule. The ever faithful **Turmeric**,with its anti-inflammatory properties, can also help reduce inflammation and damage to the stomach lining and can also be added to food.

Inflammatory bowel disease (IBD)

IBD (Inflammatory Bowel Disease) and IBS (Irritable Bowel Syndrome) are not the same condition, although they are both related to the digestive system. IBD is a chronic inflammatory condition that affects the lining of the digestive tract

The two most common types of IBD are Crohn's disease and ulcerative colitis. In these conditions, the immune system mistakenly attacks the lining of the digestive tract, causing inflammation, ulceration, and scarring. The symptoms of IBD may include abdominal pain, diarrhea, blood in the stool, fatigue, and weight loss. IBD requires medical treatment and can have serious long-term complications if left untreated.

On the other hand, IBS is a functional gastrointestinal disorder that affects the way the muscles in the digestive system work. In IBS, the muscles may contract too strongly or too weakly, causing symptoms such as abdominal pain, bloating, gas, diarrhea, or constipation.

IBS does not cause inflammation or other damage to the digestive tract, and it is not associated with an increased risk of colon cancer. IBS can be managed with lifestyle changes, such as dietary modifications and stress reduction techniques, as well as with medication in some cases.

IBS has been covered in an earlier chapter but for IBD these herbal remedies have shown promise in scientific studies but more research is needed to fully understand their effectiveness and safety for people with IBD.

Some studies have shown that curcumin, the active ingredient in **Turmeric**, may help reduce inflammation in the gut and improve symptoms of ulcerative colitis while some have suggested that **Aloe Vera, Slippery Elm** and **Boswellia** supplements or topical gels may help alleviate these symptoms.

Acid Reflux

This is covered in an earlier chapter.

Stomach upset

An upset stomach can have various causes, including infections caused by bacteria or viruses, such as gastroenteritis or food poisoning, stress, overeating, eating too quickly, consuming spicy or fatty foods, drinking too much alcohol or caffeine, and smoking.

Indigestion, also known as dyspepsia, is a type of stomach upset that can cause discomfort or pain in the upper abdomen. Other symptoms may include bloating, nausea, and a feeling of fullness after eating.

Gastroenteritis, also known as stomach flu, is a type of stomach upset caused by a viral or bacterial infection. Symptoms may include diarrhea, nausea, vomiting, abdominal cramps, and fever.

Some people may experience a stomach upset or other digestive symptoms after eating certain foods that they are intolerant to. Common food intolerances include lactose intolerance and gluten intolerance.

The symptoms of food poisoning can vary depending on the specific type of contaminant and the severity of the infection. Here are some examples of common types of food poisoning and their associated symptoms:

Salmonella is a type of bacteria that is usually found in raw or undercooked poultry, eggs, and meat, as well as in unpasteurized milk and dairy products. Symptoms of salmonella poisoning can include diarrhea, fever, abdominal cramps, and vomiting.

Campylobacter another type of bacteria, is found in raw or undercooked poultry, meat, and unpasteurized milk. Symptoms of campylobacter poisoning can include diarrhea (sometimes bloody), fever, abdominal pain and cramping, nausea, and vomiting.

E. coli is also a type of bacteria that is can be found in undercooked ground beef and contaminated produce such as lettuce and spinach. Symptoms of E. coli poisoning can include diarrhea (sometimes bloody), abdominal pain and cramping, nausea, and vomiting.

Norovirus is a type of virus that can be spread through contaminated food, water, or surfaces. Symptoms of norovirus poisoning can include diarrhea, vomiting, nausea, stomach cramps, and fever.

Listeria is a type of bacteria that can be found in a variety of foods, including deli meats, soft cheeses, and smoked seafood. Symptoms of listeria poisoning can include fever, muscle aches, nausea, and diarrhea.

If you suspect that you have food poisoning, it's important to stay hydrated and rest. In severe cases or if you are at high risk for complications (such as pregnant women or individuals with weakened immune systems), it's important to seek medical attention.

While herbal remedies may have some potential benefits for digestive health, there is limited scientific evidence to support their use specifically for treating food poisoning but **Peppermint**, **Garlic** and **Ginger** have some scientific evidence to support their use for stomach upsets in general and potentially for food poisoning.

A healthcare professional can diagnose the specific type of food poisoning that you may have, and recommend appropriate treatment.

Now that we understand some of the common causes of stomach pain and upset let's summarise some herbal remedies that can generally help alleviate the symptoms. These herbs will help with both conditions and some have been mentioned already.

One of the most effective herbal remedies is **Ginger**. Its anti-inflammatory properties help reduce inflammation in the digestive tract. Additionally, Ginger has a soothing effect on the stomach, which can help alleviate nausea and vomiting. You can consume Ginger in various forms, such as ginger tea, capsules, or fresh ginger root.

Peppermint, with its antispasmodic properties, can reduce muscle spasms in the digestive tract. This herb is especially helpful in relieving the symptoms of irritable bowel syndrome (IBS). You can consume peppermint in the form of tea or capsules.

Chamomile tea can help reduce inflammation in the digestive tract and relieve the symptoms of indigestion and acid reflux. It also has a mild sedative effect, which can help reduce anxiety and promote better sleep.

Licorice root can also help reduce inflammation in the digestive tract and protect the stomach lining from damage. Due to its soothing effect on the stomach, it can help to alleviate the symptoms of acid reflux and stomach ulcers. You can consume licorice root in the form of tea or capsules.

Fennel is an herb that can help relieve the symptoms of indigestion and bloating. Like Ginger, Fennel seeds have antispasmodic properties that can help reduce muscle spasms in the digestive tract. Additionally, fennel can also help reduce inflammation in the digestive tract and promote better digestion. You can consume Fennel in the form of tea or capsules.

thrush

THRUSH IS a common condition that affects many people, but did you know that there are different types of thrush? That's right, and knowing the difference can help you treat it more effectively.

The most common type of thrush is oral thrush, which affects the mouth and throat. It's caused by an overgrowth of a fungus called Candida, which is normally present in the mouth in small amounts. However, when the balance of bacteria and fungi in the mouth is disrupted, Candida can multiply and cause infection.

The symptoms of oral thrush include white or yellowish patches on the tongue, inside of the cheeks, or roof of the mouth, as well as soreness, redness, and difficulty swallowing. In severe cases, it can even spread to the esophagus and cause chest pain.

So, what are the best herbal remedies for oral thrush? One popular option is **Tea Tree** oil, which has antifungal properties and can help reduce the growth of Candida. You can dilute a few drops of Tea Tree oil in water and use it as a mouthwash or gargle. Another herb to consider is Garlic, which also has antifungal properties and can be consumed raw or in supplement form.

But what about vaginal thrush? This type of thrush affects the genital area and is caused by an overgrowth of Candida in the vagina. It's more common in women, but men can also develop it. The symptoms of vaginal thrush include itching, burning, and discharge that may be thick and white.

If you're looking for herbal remedies for vaginal thrush, one option is probiotics. Probiotics are live bacteria and yeasts that are good for your health, which can restore the balance of bacteria and fungi in your body. You can take probiotic supplements or eat foods that are high in probiotics, such as yogurt or kefir.

Another herb to consider for vaginal thrush is **Calendula**. This is a type of marigold that has antifungal properties that can reduce inflammation and itching. You can make a tea or infusion with calendula flowers and use it as a wash or soak for the affected area.

Lastly, let's talk about thrush in babies. Thrush can affect infants, especially those who are breastfeeding. It's caused by the same fungus that causes oral thrush in adults, which can cause white patches on the tongue and inside of the mouth, as well as feeding difficulties.

If you're looking for herbal remedies for thrush in babies, one option is Coconut oil. It has antifungal properties and can be applied to the affected area to help reduce the growth of Candida. Another herb to consider is **Chamomile**, which has anti-inflammatory properties and can help soothe irritated skin. You can make a tea with chamomile flowers and use it as a wash for your baby's mouth or skin.

Thrush can be an uncomfortable and unpleasant condition, whether you're dealing with oral thrush, vaginal thrush, or thrush in babies, there are herbs that can help reduce inflammation, soothe irritated skin, and reduce the growth of Candida.

forty-nine
thyroid

THE THYROID IS a small gland located in the neck that plays a vital role in regulating our metabolism and hormone balance. When the thyroid is not functioning properly, it can lead to a variety of symptoms including weight changes, fatigue, and mood changes.

There are a number of causes that can lead to thyroid problems including, for women, the menopause. During menopause, the levels of estrogen and progesterone decrease and this reduction in estrogen levels can cause the thyroid gland to slow down, leading to hypothyroidism (see below).

Genetics also plays a role and if thyroid problems run in your family, you may be more likely to develop them.

If you have had radiation therapy to your neck or chest, you may be at an increased risk of developing thyroid problems and certain medications, such as lithium, can affect thyroid function.

Finally, autoimmune disorders, such as Hashimoto's thyroiditis and Graves' disease, can all cause thyroid problems.

The most common thyroid problems are hypothyroidism and hyper-thyroidism.

Hypothyroidism

Hypothyroidism is a condition in which the thyroid gland does not produce enough thyroid hormones. These hormones are essential for regulating many of the body's functions, including metabolism, growth and development, and the function of the nervous system. When there is not enough thyroid hormone in the body, many bodily functions can slow down, leading to a variety of symptoms.

There are several different causes of hypothyroidism. The most common cause is an autoimmune disorder called Hashimoto's thyroiditis. In this condition, the body's immune system attacks the thyroid gland, causing inflammation and damage that can impair its ability to produce hormones.

Other causes of hypothyroidism include damage to the thyroid gland from radiation treatment, surgery to remove the thyroid gland, the menopause or certain medications. These include Lithium, used to treat bipolar disorder and Amiodarone which is used to treat heart arrhythmias. It contains iodine, which can cause either hypothyroidism or hyperthyroidism, depending on the person.

Interferon alpha is a medication used to treat hepatitis C and certain types of cancer. It can cause autoimmune thyroid disease, which can lead to hypothyroidism. Tyrosine kinase inhibitors, can interfere with the production of thyroid hormones, leading to hypothyroidism and these are also used to treat cancer and some anti-seizure medications, such as carbamazepine and phenytoin, can interfere with the absorption of thyroid hormones, leading to hypothyroidism.

Not everyone who takes these medications will develop hypothyroidism. However, if you are taking any of these medications and are experiencing symptoms of hypothyroidism it is important to talk to your doctor.

The symptoms of hypothyroidism can vary depending on the severity of the condition and how long it has been present. In some cases, symptoms may be mild and may not be immediately noticeable, while in other cases they can be severe and have a significant impact on quality of life.

One of the most common symptoms of hypothyroidism is fatigue. You would often feel tired and sluggish, even after getting enough sleep and may also experience weakness in their muscles, making it difficult to perform everyday activities.

Another common symptom of hypothyroidism is weight gain. You may find it difficult to lose weight or may gain weight even when you are not consuming excess calories. This is because the body's metabolism slows down when there is not enough thyroid hormone in the body, making it more difficult to burn calories.

Other symptoms of hypothyroidism can include dry skin and hair, hair loss, cold intolerance, constipation, depression, and difficulty concentrating. In severe cases, hypothyroidism can lead to a condition called myxedema, which can cause extreme fatigue, confusion, and even coma.

While conventional medical treatments for hypothyroidism typically involve thyroid hormone replacement therapy, there are also many herbal remedies that may help to support thyroid function and alleviate some of the symptoms.

One herb that may be helpful for supporting thyroid function is **Ashwagandha**. Ashwagandha is an adaptogenic herb that is known for its ability to help the body cope with stress. It may also help to regulate thyroid function by balancing levels of thyroid hormones in the body. In one study, Ashwagandha supplementation was found to improve thyroid function in people with subclinical hypothyroidism, a condition in which thyroid hormone levels are slightly low but not yet low enough to warrant conventional treatment.

Another herb that may be beneficial for hypothyroidism is **Bladder-wrack.** Bladderwrack is a type of seaweed that is rich in iodine, a mineral that is essential for thyroid function. In areas where iodine deficiency is common, Bladderwrack has traditionally been used to prevent and treat hypothyroidism. However, it's important to note that excessive iodine intake can also be harmful, so it's best to talk with a healthcare professional before using Bladderwrack or any other iodine-containing herbs.

Guggul is yet another herb that may be helpful. It is a resin that is extracted from the mukul myrrh tree and has traditionally been used in Ayurvedic medicine to treat a variety of conditions, including hypothyroidism. Some studies have suggested that Guggul may help to stimulate thyroid function by increasing the production of thyroid hormones.

Finally, **Holy Basil**, also known as Tulsi, may also be helpful.

Hyperthyroidism

Hyperthyroidism, also known as overactive thyroid, is as you might expect the opposite of hypothyroidism, and it is when the thyroid gland produces an excessive amount of thyroid hormone.

Symptoms of hyperthyroidism can vary from person to person, but some of the most common include weight loss, increased appetite, rapid heartbeat, sweating, nervousness, fatigue, muscle weakness, and difficulty sleeping. Other symptoms can include tremors, frequent bowel movements, and changes in menstrual cycles.

The causes of hyperthyroidism can also vary, but the most common cause is an autoimmune disorder called Graves' disease. This occurs when the immune system mistakenly attacks the thyroid gland, causing it to produce too much hormone. Other causes of hyperthyroidism include thyroid nodules, thyroiditis (inflammation of the thyroid gland), and taking too much thyroid hormone medication.

If left untreated, hyperthyroidism can lead to more severe health problems, such as heart palpitations, osteoporosis, and even a life-threatening condition called thyroid storm. It is essential to see a healthcare provider if you experience any of the symptoms of hyperthyroidism to get proper diagnosis and treatment.

Herbal remedies can be a helpful addition to conventional treatment for hyperthyroidism. Here are some herbs that may be beneficial:

Bugleweed is a natural herb that can help reduce the amount of thyroid hormone produced by the thyroid gland, making it useful in managing symptoms of hyperthyroidism.

Lemon balm, known for its calming properties, can help reduce anxiety and nervousness associated with hyperthyroidism. It also has antiviral properties and can help boost the immune system.

Motherwort is can regulate the heart and nervous system. which helps to reduce the heart palpitations and anxiety associated with hyperthyroidism. It also has anti-inflammatory properties and so it can help reduce inflammation in the thyroid gland.

Ashwagandha, once more, helps to reduce stress and anxiety associated with its anti-inflammatory properties it cab help reduce inflammation in the thyroid gland.

It is important to note that while these herbs can be beneficial for managing symptoms of hyperthyroidism, they should be used under the guidance of a healthcare provider. Some herbs can interact with medications, so it is important to discuss any herbal remedies with your healthcare provider before using them.

A natural remedy that may be helpful for hyperthyroidism is a tea made from a combination of these herbs. Here is a recipe for a hyper-thyroidism tea:

Ingredients:

- 1 teaspoon bugleweed
- 1 teaspoon lemon balm
- 1 teaspoon motherwort
- 1 teaspoon ashwagandha
- 4 cups of water

Directions:

1. In a medium saucepan, bring 4 cups of water to a boil.
2. Add the bugleweed, lemon balm, motherwort, and ashwagandha to the water.
3. Reduce heat to a simmer and let the herbs steep for 15-20 minutes.
4. Remove from heat and strain the tea into a mug.
5. Drink 2-3 cups per day.

fifty
toothache

THERE ARE several reasons why you may be suffering from toothache. You may have had a wisdom tooth break the skin, or you might have cracked or damaged a tooth. There is also the possibility that you have tooth decay or an abscess.

The first thing that you should do is book an appointment with your dentist. You cannot use herbal medicine as a replacement for dentistry! However, if your toothache is due to wisdom teeth, you will need some pain relief, as getting your wisdom teeth removed can take a while.

The goal of herbal medicine here is to numb the area so that there is less pain and to reduce inflammation. You can use a **Peppermint** tea bag to reduce pain in the gums. Soak it in cold water, then place it over the tooth and gum. Peppermint has a natural pain-relieving and antibacterial effect.

Cloves have been used for toothache for centuries and are still recommended by many dentists as a form of pain relief for toothache.

Clove tea is made from the dried buds of the clove plant. It has a warm, spicy flavor and has natural pain-relieving and antibacterial properties.

It is also believed to have digestive and immune-boosting benefits.

Instructions for clove tea

- Place the clove buds in a tea infuser or wrap them in a piece of cheesecloth.
- Place the tea infuser or cheesecloth with the clove buds in a cup.
- Pour the boiling water over the clove buds.
- Allow the tea to steep for 5-10 minutes.
- Remove the tea infuser or cheesecloth with the clove buds.
- Drink the tea while it is still warm.

Use a clove oil extract to reduce inflammation and provide an antiseptic solution. Place some drops onto a cotton bud and then rub gently around the gums and tooth. You can also add clove oil to water to create a mouthwash. To make your own clove oil, crush 2-3 cloves and add to live oil - you can do this in an egg cup!

If you want to reduce the risk of tooth decay, then create a mouthwash using **Thyme** oil extract. Thyme offers antibacterial properties that can help protect your teeth from tooth decay in the first place.

Another option is to create a **Garlic** paste using a garlic clove and some salt. Then apply this to the tooth and gums. You may want to keep a distance from friends and family after rubbing raw garlic in your mouth, but the results will be worth it.

You can of course make a tea from Chamomile, Peppermint and Ginger. While Chamomile can soothe the pain, Ginger also has a natural pain-relieving effect.

Salt water is a very well-known method for disinfecting your teeth, though whether salt is considered a herbal remedy is up to you to decide.

Adding a couple of pinches of salt to a cup of warm water then swilling it around your mouth is particularly effective for keeping your teeth free from infection when suffering from wisdom tooth growth.

Native Americans in used thorns from the **Prickly Elder tree** as a form of pain relief for toothache. It was also used as a medicine during the American Civil War. It has been shown to provide antimicrobial properties and may be an effective weapon against antibiotic-resistant bacteria.

Remember, prevention is better than treatment when it comes to toothache. As well as regular dental appointments and cleaning your teeth regularly, you can use cloves or thyme mouthwashes to disinfect your teeth and protect them from decay.

Abscess

An abscess is a painful collection of pus, usually caused by a bacterial infection. The intention of any treatment is to drain the abscess and this is what garlic can effectively do. It is both antibacterial and antimicrobial. I know this, because I had an abscess on my gum recently. It's also remarkably easy, painless and fast.

Chop up and crush your garlic and place a small amount on a cloth to make a mini-poultice. Dab this onto your abscess. You will know if you have too much garlic because you won't be able to touch it onto your abscess - it will sting and it will feel very hot. Once you have the right amount, try to hold it there for a few seconds and then re-apply a few times over a period of around 10 minutes.

You should feel your abscess getting smaller within an hour and gone completely within 6 to 8 hours. As someone who uses herbs all the time, it was the first time I had ever tried this remedy. I also had a cup of Sage tea following the garlic dabbing. Even I was amazed at the result!

fifty-one
urinary tract infection (uti)

UTIs ARE a common condition that affects both men and women, and they can be caused by a variety of factors that are detailed below.

The most common cause of a UTI is a bacterial infection. This occurs when bacteria, usually E. coli, enters the urinary tract through the urethra and starts to multiply. The body reacts to this invasion by producing white blood cells, which can lead to inflammation and discomfort.

Uva Ursi, also known as bearberry, has been used by Native American tribes for centuries to treat urinary tract infections and other urinary problems. It contains compounds called arbutin and hydroquinone, which are known for their antibacterial properties.

Cranberry is another useful herb for UTIs, as it contains compounds called proanthocyanidins that prevent bacteria from sticking to the walls of the urinary tract. It is important to note that it is only effective in preventing bacterial infections, not treating them once they occur.

Goldenseal is a third option, as it contains the alkaloid berberine, which has been shown to have antibacterial properties.

<u>Recipe</u>: To make a tea, combine 1 tsp of dried uva ursi leaves, 1 tsp of dried cranberry, and 1 tsp of dried goldenseal root in a teapot. Pour 8 oz of boiling water over the herbs and let steep for 10-15 minutes. Strain and drink 2-3 cups a day.

Do not use goldenseal if you are pregnant or have high blood pressure.

Another common cause of UTIs is a yeast infection. This occurs when the yeast Candida overgrows in the urinary tract. Yeast infections are more common in women and can be caused by a variety of factors, including antibiotics, hormonal changes, and weakened immune systems. We cover yeast infections in a later chapter, but we have added some additional herbs here.

Garlic is a potent herb used to treat yeast infections because it contains compounds called allicin and ajoene, which have antifungal properties.

Pau d'Arco is another herb that is effective against yeast infections, as it contains compounds called lapachol and beta-lapachone, both of which have antifungal properties. Oregon grape root is a third option, it contains the alkaloid berberine which has been shown to have antifungal properties.

<u>Recipe:</u> To make a tea, combine 1 tsp of chopped garlic, 1 tsp of dried pau d'arco bark, and 1 tsp of dried oregon grape root in a teapot. Pour 8 oz of boiling water over the herbs and let steep for 10-15 minutes. Strain and drink 2-3 cups a day.

Do not use garlic if you are taking blood-thinning medication or have a bleeding disorder.

Kidney stones can also cause a UTI. These are hard deposits of minerals and salts that form in the kidneys. When these stones pass through the urinary tract, they can cause pain, discomfort, and infection.

Chanca piedra is a powerful herb that is used to treat kidney stones because it contains compounds that help to break down the stones and prevent them from forming.

Dandelion root is another effective herb against kidney stones, as it helps to flush out the urinary tract and prevent the stones from forming .

Horsetail is a third option, as it is rich in silica, which helps to strengthen the urinary tract and prevent the formation of kidney stones.

Recipe: To make a tea, combine 1 tsp of dried chanca piedra, 1 tsp of dried dandelion root, and 1 tsp of dried horsetail in a teapot. Pour 8 oz of boiling water over the herbs and let steep for 10-15 minutes. Strain and drink 2-3 cups a day.

Note: Do not use horsetail if you are pregnant or have low potassium levels.

As ever, it is important to consult with a healthcare provider before using any herbal remedies, especially if you are pregnant or have a medical condition. Stay healthy and happy!

fifty-two
wounds

THE MOST IMPORTANT thing that you can do when wounded is to first assess the damage. How large is the wound? Is it something that can be treated at home, or do you need to see a doctor?

If the former, then there are a number of herbs that you can use in treatment. But the most important thing to do is first clean the wound with water and to change the dressings regularly. Here are five herbal remedies that you can use to treat minor wounds.

- **Eucalyptus** – A 2002 study looked into the effects of a tincture of eucalyptus on wound healing. It found significant healing properties in wounds treated by a few drops of eucalyptus. Adding your tincture to bandages and changing them regularly appears to be an effective way to treat wounds.
- **Aloe Vera**- A commonly used herbal remedy for wounds, aloe vera works by reducing inflammation and accelerates wound healing. However, be careful when using on serious burn as it can actually react badly to burned tissue. Aloe vera may also offer an antibacterial benefit for wounds.

- **Chamomile** – As with aloe vera, chamomile works by decreasing inflammation in a wound, particularly infected wounds. An essential oil or tincture of chamomile applied to a bandage is a good idea for wound healing.
- **Rosemary** – Rosemary provides both anti-inflammatory and antimicrobial properties, meaning that it can reduce inflammation and reduce the risk of infection when applied to wounds. Tinctures of rosemary applied to a clean bandage may speed up the healing process.
- **Curcumin** – This is the active ingredient found in turmeric; when applied as an ointment to wounds, curcumin can increase collagen production, which is crucial for wound healing.

One form of wound care that is found in many cultures is **Honey**. Not only can it reduce inflammation, but it also has antimicrobial properties, reducing the risk of infection. The trick with honey is to apply it to the dressing first, rather than placing it straight on the wound.

It is often recommended to mix honey with other ingredients when you make a poultice or dressing for wound healing. You can try this recipe that uses honey as part of a poultice with additional ingredients to make it more effective:

Ingredients:

- 1 tablespoon honey
- 1 tablespoon coconut oil or olive oil
- 1-2 tablespoons flour or cornstarch
- Warm water
- A clean cloth or gauze

Instructions:

1. Mix the honey, oil, and flour or cornstarch together in a small bowl to form a paste.
2. Clean the wound thoroughly with warm water and mild soap, and pat it dry with a clean towel.
3. Apply a thin layer of the honey mixture onto the wound. Make sure the paste covers the entire wound.
4. Place the clean cloth or gauze over the honey paste and press it gently into place.
5. Leave the poultice on for 30 minutes to an hour.
6. Remove the poultice and clean the wound again with warm water.
7. Repeat the process once or twice a day until the wound has healed.

As with any wound, assess it first, and get a doctor to look at it if you think that the wound may be difficult to treat at home. You can then inform the doctor that you want to use honey to treat the wound. In a perfect world, they will understand immediately and then show you how best to apply it.

You may also want to consider a poultice with **OMT Blue clay**. A 2018 study in the International Journal of Antimicrobial Agents took a look at OMT Blue clay, a type of healing clay that is often used in herbal medicine.

The study found that it had incredible antimicrobial effects, protecting wounds against staphylococci, streptococci, and Enterobacteriaceae infections.

Other poultice ingredients that could work well are **Ginger**, **Eucalyptus**, **Garlic**, and **Turmeric**.

You can also consider using food to help with wound healing. **Ginger, garlic, Turmeric**, and **Rosemary** can all be cooked in different dishes. Each will offer some help with wound healing and reducing infection risk.

Sleeping 8 hours a night and taking part in gentle exercise (walking, yoga) can help speed up wound healing, particularly when combined with the herbal remedies and poultices described above. Sleep is when your body begins to heal, and exercise can increase blood flow which will help the wound to heal.

fifty-three
yeast infection

YEAST INFECTIONS ARE a common problem among women, but they can also occur in men. They are due to an overgrowth of a type of fungus called Candida which causes an imbalance of the natural bacteria and yeast in the body.

This imbalance can be caused by a variety of factors, including a weakened immune system, antibiotics, pregnancy, diabetes, and tight clothing. In this chapter, we will explore the most common causes of a yeast infection and the best herbal remedies to treat each cause.

Antibiotics

Antibiotic use and overuse is one of the most common causes of yeast infections because they kill the beneficial bacteria in the body that keep the Candida fungus in check, leading to an overgrowth of yeast. The body reacts to this overgrowth by causing inflammation, itching, and burning in the affected area.

Calendula can help to reduce inflammation and itching caused by a yeast infection and it has antifungal properties that can help to kill the Candida fungus.

You can make a tea by steeping one teaspoon of dried calendula flowers in one cup of boiling water for 10-15 minutes. You can drink the tea or apply it to the affected area using a cotton ball.

In a study published in the Journal of Antimicrobial Chemotherapy, researchers found that **Garlic** extract had strong antifungal activity against Candida albicans, the fungus that causes most yeast infections.

To use Garlic for a yeast infection, you can crush a few cloves of garlic and apply it directly to the affected area. Alternatively, you can take garlic supplements.

Echinacea can help to boost the immune system and prevent yeast infections caused by antibiotics. It also has antifungal properties that can help to kill the Candida fungus.

To use Echinacea, you can make a tea by steeping one teaspoon of dried echinacea root in one cup of boiling water for 10-15 minutes. Drink the tea or apply it to the affected area using a cotton ball.

Pregnancy

Hormonal changes during pregnancy can alter the balance of bacteria and yeast in the body, leading to too much yeast. The body reacts to this overgrowth by causing itching, burning, and discharge in the vaginal area. Before you use any herbs while pregnant it is always recommended to consult with a health professional.

Chamomile has anti-inflammatory properties and can help to reduce inflammation and itching caused and has antifungal properties that can help to kill the Candida fungus.

To prepare Chamomile, you can make a tea by steeping one teaspoon of dried chamomile flowers in one cup of boiling water for 10-15 minutes. You can drink the tea or apply it to the affected area using a cotton ball.

Yogurt is a natural probiotic that can help to restore the natural balance of bacteria and yeast in the body. It contains live cultures of Lactobacillus acidophilus, which can help to prevent yeast infections. To use yogurt for a yeast infection, you can apply plain, unsweetened yogurt directly to the affected area.

In a study published in the Journal of Obstetrics and Gynaecology Research, researchers found that topical application of **Tea Tree Oil** was effective in treating vaginal yeast infections.

It is an essential oil that has antifungal properties and can help to kill the Candida fungus. However, it should be used with caution during pregnancy as it can cause skin irritation.

To use tea tree oil for a yeast infection, you can mix a few drops with a carrier oil, such as coconut oil, and apply it to the affected area.

Diabetes

People with diabetes are more prone to yeast infections because high blood sugar levels can promote the growth of yeast. Yeast infections in people with diabetes can affect various parts of the body, including the skin, nails, and mouth.

Herbal remedies for yeast infections caused by diabetes are outlined below.

In a study published in the Journal of Ethnopharmacology, researchers found that **Cinnamon** has antifungal activity against Candida albicans, the fungus that causes most yeast infections. Cinnamon can also help to reduce blood sugar levels in people with diabetes. Don't use cinnamon if you are pregnant.

To use Cinnamon for a yeast infection, you can make a tea by steeping one cinnamon stick in one cup of boiling water for 10-15 minutes. You can drink the tea or apply it to the affected area using a cotton ball.

Oregano with its antifungal properties can help to kill the Candida fungus. It also has antibacterial and anti-inflammatory properties that can help to reduce inflammation and itching.

To use Oregano for a yeast infection, you can make a tea by following the same method as Chamomile, Calendula and Echinacea.

Aloe vera is a plant that also has anti-inflammatory and antifungal properties that can help to reduce inflammation and itching caused by a yeast infection. It can also help to soothe the skin.

To use Aloe Vera for a yeast infection, you can apply the gel from a fresh aloe vera leaf to the affected area.

Herbal remedies can be effective in treating yeast infections by reducing inflammation and itching, killing the Candida fungus, and restoring the natural balance of bacteria and yeast in the body. Always look out for a herb with antifungal and anti-inflammatory properties.

Yeast infections can also cause an Urinary Tract Infection (see the chapter on UTI).

fifty-four
precautions

HERBS ARE POWERFUL, and many, if not most, need to be taken with respect. Here we aim to details some herbs and the precautions that you may need to consider as an example of what to look out for and to impress upon you that knowing the downsides of any herb is important.

It goes without saying that you should consult with a healthcare provider if you are taking any medications or are pregnant or breast-feeding before taking any herbs. Always follow dosage instructions carefully, and monitor for any potential side effects. If you experience any adverse effects while using a herb, you should stop using it immediately and talk to your healthcare provider.

While herbs are generally considered safe, it is important to use them with caution and to be aware of any potential risks or interactions.

Here are some precautions and health considerations to keep in mind when using some popular herbs. This is not an exhaustive list and while it provides examples, it should underline that you need to check which herbs you are using, or plan to use.

Aloe Vera

While Aloe Vera has many beneficial properties and is often used topically to help soothe and heal skin irritations, it is not recommended for internal consumption. The gel found inside the aloe vera plant contains a compound called aloin, which can have laxative effects and may cause diarrhea or other digestive issues if consumed in large amounts. In addition, some studies have suggested that consuming Aloe Vera may be associated with an increased risk of certain health problems, such as kidney disease or electrolyte imbalances. Therefore, it is generally recommended to avoid consuming Aloe Vera internally, unless under the supervision of a healthcare professional who can advise on the appropriate dosage and potential risks. If you are looking to incorporate Aloe Vera into your diet, it is best to stick with products that are specifically formulated for internal consumption.

Basil

Basil should be used with caution if you are taking blood thinners or antiplatelet drugs.

Ashwagandha

Ashwagandha may interact with certain medications for thyroid disorders and those that suppress the immune system.

Calendula

Some people may experience an allergic reaction to calendula, so it is important to do a patch test before using it on a larger area of skin when using topically.

Catnip

Excessive use can lead to vomiting. Not recommended for use in pregnant women.

Chamomile

Roman chamomile has a greater chance of causing an allergic reaction than German chamomile and those sensitive to ragweed may have severe reactions to this plant. Symptoms of an allergic reaction may include skin rash, itching, and difficulty breathing.

It is a natural blood thinner and which means it impact blood-thinning medications, such as warfarin, and it can have a mild sedative effect. It may also drowsiness when combined with other sedative medications, such as benzodiazepines or opioids.

Lastly, chamomile may have uterine-stimulating effects and should be avoided during pregnancy.

Cilantro/Coriander

Cilantro and coriander come from the same plant and some people may be allergic to cilantro, and coriander may interact with some blood thinners and antidiabetic drugs.

Cinnamon

Not suitable for use when suffering from fever, blood in your urine, excessive dryness, dry stools, hemorrhoids, or while nursing or pregnant.

Dandellion

Professional medical advice or guidance is advised for people with gallstones or structured bile ducts. Excessive use may cause allergic reactions, abdominal problems, heartburn, nausea, or loose stools. Possible worsened symptoms in gastric hyperacidity.

Elderberry

Although Elderberry is generally safe there are a few conditions when is should not be used. Because it stimulates the immune system people with autoimmune disorders such as lupus, rheumatoid arthritis, or multiple sclerosis or those taking immunosuppressive drugs used to treat conditions such as organ transplants should not use it.

There is also limited research on the safety of elderberry during pregnancy and breastfeeding, so it's best to avoid it or use it with caution under the guidance of a healthcare provider.

Finally young children including those under a year old should not be given Elderberry. This is because their immune systems are still developing and may not be able to handle the stimulation from elderberry.

Finally, if you have an allergy to any plants in the Elder family, you should avoid this member of the family.

Fennel

People with kidney disease should also be cautious when using fennel, as it can exacerbate the condition. Not to be used in conjunction with tamoxifen, estrogen, contraceptives, or ciprofloxacin.

Garlic

Don't use garlic if you are taking blood-thinning medication or have a bleeding disorder. High doses of garlic can cause digestive upset in some people.

Ginkgo biloba

Ginkgo can interact blood thinners and antidepressants.

Ginger

Ginger in not suitable for use when suffering from hyperacidity, peptic ulcers, or any hot inflammatory conditions. Not to be used in conjunction with blood-thinning drugs. A maximum of one gram is recommended for pregnant women. **Goldenseal**

One of the main concerns is that goldenseal can disrupt the balance of bacteria in the gut which can lead to digestive problems, such as bloating, gas, and diarrhea. In addition, goldenseal can also reduce the absorption of certain nutrients, such as iron, calcium, and vitamin B, which can lead to deficiencies over time.

Another potential risk is that it can interact with certain medications. For example, it can increase the effects of sedatives and blood pressure medications, and decrease the effectiveness of some antibiotics and birth control pills.

Finally, there is some concern that long-term use of goldenseal may cause liver damage, although this has not been definitively proven.

Horsetail

Avoid horsetail if you are pregnant or have low potassium levels.

Lavender

Lavender should not be taken internally during pregnancy or breast-feeding, and it can interfere with other medications, including sedatives.

Lemon Balm

Lemon balm is generally safe for most people but it may interact with thyroid medications and sedatives. Because it can reduce thyroid functions, it's not recommended for individuals with underactive thyroids.

Licorice

Licorice root contains compounds called glycyrrhizic acid and glycyrrhetinic acid, which can cause a range of side effects, and can lead to high blood pressure, low potassium levels, and an increased risk of heart disease. In addition, long-term or excessive use of licorice root can lead to fluid retention, swelling, and headaches.

Another potential risk is that licorice root can interact with certain medications. For example, it can increase the effects of corticosteroids and digoxin, and decrease the effectiveness of some blood pressure medications and diuretics.

Finally, Licorice root can also have estrogen-like effects, which can be a concern for women who have a history of hormone-sensitive cancers or other conditions. Therefore, it is important to use Licorice root with caution in these situations, and to refer to a healthcare provider before using it.

Marshmallow Root

Some people may experience allergic reactions to marshmallow root, particularly if they are allergic to other plants in the mallow family.

Signs of an allergic reaction may include hives, rash, itching, difficulty breathing, or swelling of the face, lips, tongue, or throat. If you experience any of these symptoms while using marshmallow root, you should stop using it immediately and seek medical attention.

Marshmallow root can also interact with certain medications, particularly those that are broken down by the liver. It can also decrease the absorption of some medications if taken at the same time.

People with diabetes should use it with caution and under the guidance of a healthcare provider because it can lower blood sugar levels. It can also cause gastrointestinal side effects such as nausea, diarrhea, or stomach upset in some people. This means that it's important to start with a low dose and gradually increase it over time to minimize the risk of gastrointestinal side effects.

Mint/Peppermint

Peppermint can interact with blood thinners and antidiabetic drugs. Nursing mothers can use it, but in moderation. In excess amounts it can cause drying of the breast milk. and pregnant women should only have up to two cups a day. Not for people with gallstone problems, yin deficiency, and cold conditions.

Nettle

Ingesting nettle may cause mild side effects such as stomach upset, diarrhea, and sweating. Additionally, nettle could interact with certain medications, including blood thinners, blood pressure medications, and diabetes medications.

It can also cause an allergic reaction, particularly those with a history of hay fever or allergies to plants. Symptoms of an allergic reaction may include itching, rash, and difficulty breathing. If you experience any of these symptoms while using nettle, you should stop using it immediately and seek medical attention.

Rosemary

Rosemary can have an effect on with certain blood thinners.

Saffron

Saffron may effect the efficiency of antidepressants and blood thinners.

Thyme

Thyme can interact with blood thinners and antidiabetic drugs.

Herbs to use with caution

Here is a list of some herbs that you may want to use with caution:

- Comfrey, Coltsfoot, Kava and Pennyroyal have all been linked to liver damage and Pennyroyal may also have a toxic effect on the heart.
- Sassafras contains safrole, which has been linked to cancer in animals.
- Lobelia is a herb that can be toxic in high doses.
- Ephedra (also known as ma huang), Yohimbe and Khathas have been linked to increased blood pressure and heart rate, and may increase the risk of heart attack and stroke.
- Angelica is a herb that has been linked to irregular heart rhythm.
- Aconite and Foxglove can have a toxic effects on the heart.

fifty-five
conclusion

As we reach the end of this book, I hope that you have gained a deeper appreciation for the power of herbal medicine. Throughout the pages of this book, we have explored some of the science behind its effectiveness, and the specific herbs and natural remedies that can be used to treat common illnesses. Of the herbs listed in the pages of this book, there are many others that could take their place.

One of the key reasons why herbs are so effective in promoting health and healing is that they work in harmony with our bodies. Many herbs contain natural compounds that have medicinal properties, such as anti-inflammatory, antimicrobial, and antioxidant effects. When we consume these herbs, these natural compounds interact with our body's cells and tissues to promote healing and restore balance.

For example, when we consume herbs such as Echinacea and Elderberry, they can help boost our immune system's ability to fight off infections such as colds and flu. Other herbs such as Ginger and Peppermint can help soothe digestive issues by reducing inflammation and relaxing the muscles in the digestive tract.

Many herbs also have adaptogenic properties, meaning they can help the body adapt to stress and support overall health and wellbeing. Adaptogenic herbs such as Ashwagandha and Holy Basil can help reduce stress and anxiety, improve mood, and promote better sleep.

In addition to using herbs for healing, I encourage you to incorporate herbs into your daily life in other ways. Cook with fresh herbs to add flavor and nutrition to your meals, drink herbal teas to promote relaxation and hydration, and, of course, create herbal remedies to keep on hand for common ailments.

And remember, herbal medicine is not a one-size-fits-all solution. What works for one person may not work for another. It's important to listen to your body, trust your intuition, and experiment with different herbs and remedies to find what works best for you.

While herbs can be effective in treating common illnesses, they are not a cure-all solution. Herbal remedies should be used in conjunction with a healthy diet, regular exercise, and other lifestyle factors that contribute to overall health and wellbeing.

I hope that this book has inspired you to continue your journey into the world of herbal medicine. By using herbs to promote our health and wellbeing, we are not only improving our own lives, but we are also helping to create a healthier, more sustainable world for future generations. Let us continue to harness the power of nature and embrace the healing power of herbs.

As with any form of medicine, it's important to use herbs safely and responsibly.

fifty-six
leave a review

THANK you for reading this book and I sincerely hope that you found it valuable. I would be eternally grateful if you would take just a few seconds to leave a review. You can leave a star rating or add some words.

So let me ask you this question. If it cost you nothing to share information with a struggling individual whom you don't personally know, would you do it? This person may have much in common with you, and this person, like most, judges a book by its reviews.

If you perceive this book as a valuable resource, would you take less than 60 seconds to leave an honest review? This act of kindness costs you nothing and could really help someone on their road to discovery. All with a review.

You are welcome join our private facebook group and join those on the herbal journey!

https://www.facebook.com/groups/herbalremediesandhealth/

more from goldberry hill

Grow Your Own Herbal Medicine

How and why medicinal herbs work and how to use them. Growing guide for 21 ideal herbs to begin your magical healing garden.

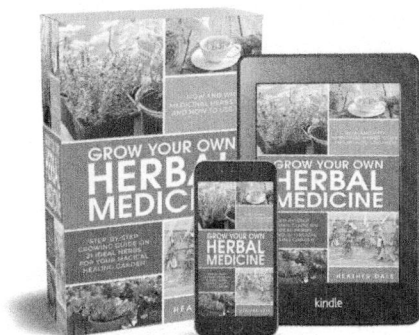

Herbal Remedies for Health and Healing For Beginners

Understand and discover the Power of Ancient Traditions for Natural Remedies for Modern Wellbeing

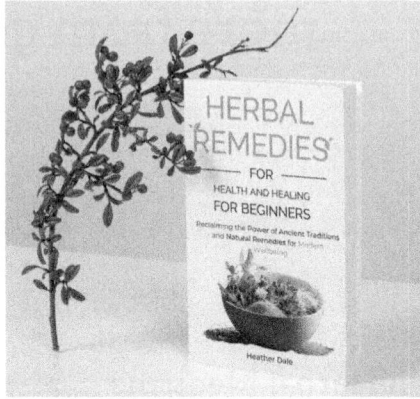

references

Understanding Herbal Remedies (Goldberry Hill)

Grow Your Own Medicinal Herbs (Goldberry Hill)

Discover the Power of Magic Tea (Goldberry Hill)

National Institute of Diabetes and Digestive and Kidney Diseases. (2021). Irritable bowel syndrome (IBS). Retrieved from https://www.niddk.nih.gov/health-information/digestive-diseases/irritable-bowel-syndrome

Supplement and Herb Guide for Arthritis Symptoms | Arthritis Foundation (no date). Available at: https://www.arthritis.org/health-wellness/treatment/complementary-therapies/supplements-and-vitamins/supplement-and-herb-guide-for-arthritis-symptoms.

Chey, W. D., Kurlander, J., & Eswaran, S. (2015). Irritable bowel syndrome: a clinical review. Jama, 313(9), 949-958.

Ford, A. C., Harris, L. A., & Lacy, B. E. (2018). Systematic review with meta-analysis: the efficacy of prebiotics, probiotics, synbiotics and antibiotics in irritable bowel syndrome. Alimentary pharmacology & therapeutics, 48(10), 1044-1060.

Khodadadi, H., & Asadolahi, M. (2021). The therapeutic effects of Curcuma longa L. extract on irritable bowel syndrome: a systematic review and meta-analysis. BMC complementary medicine and therapies, 21(1), 1-16.

Honey as a topical treatment for wounds" by C. Allen Hanberg, DPM, in Podiatry Today (2011): https://www.podiatrytoday.com/honey-topical-treatment-wounds

"Honey for wound care: A review" by M. Subrahmanyam, in World Journal of Clinical Cases (2015): https://www.ncbi.nlm.nih.gov/pmc/articles/PMC4300500/

"Honey for Wound Healing, Ulcers, and Burns; Data Supporting Its Use in Clinical Practice" by Stefan Bogdanov, in Alternative Medicine Review (2008): https://www.ncbi.nlm.nih.gov/pmc/articles/PMC2868613/

Friedrich, J., & logical, B. (2010). Green tea in dermatology. Journal of drugs in dermatology : JDD, 9(7), 753-759.)

Thammaraks, K., & Asawanonda, P. (2012). Topical green tea extract for the treatment of acne vulgaris: a randomized, double-blind, controlled trial. International journal of dermatology, 51(12), 1480-1484.)

Obón, C., Rivera, D., Fonollá, E., Alcaraz, F., & Attieh, L. (2021). A Comparison Study on Traditional Mixtures of Herbal Teas Used in Eastern Mediterranean Area. *Frontiers in Pharmacology*, 12. https://doi.org/10.3389/fphar.2021.632692

A Brief History of Skincare Through the Ages. (2019, January 14). INB Medical. Retrieved January 13, 2022, from https://www.inbmedical.com/the-evolving-role-of-skincare

OA, E., & AMA, E. (2016). Medicinal Plants and Addiction Treatment. *Medicinal & Aromatic Plants*, 05(04).https://doi.org/10.4172/2167-0412.1000260

Keefe, J. R., Mao, J. J., Soeller, I., Li, Q. S., & Amsterdam, J. D. (2016). Short-term open-label chamomile (Matricaria chamomilla L.) therapy of moderate to severe generalized anxiety disorder. *Phytomedicine*, 23(14), 1699–1705. https://doi.org/10.1016/j.phymed.2016.10.013

Shishehbor, F., Rezaeyan Safar, M., Rajaei, E., & Haghighizadeh, M. H. (2018). Cinnamon Consumption Improves Clinical Symptoms and Inflammatory Markers in Women With Rheumatoid Arthritis. *Journal of the American College of Nutrition*, 37(8), 685–690. https://doi.org/10.1080/07315724.2018.1460733

Uehleke, B., Müller, J., Stange, R., Kelber, O., & Melzer, J. (2013). Willow bark extract STW 33-I in the long-term treatment of outpatients with rheumatic pain mainly osteoarthritis or back pain. *Phytomedicine*, 20(11), 980–984. https://doi.org/10.1016/j.phymed.2013.03.023

Krikorian, R., Shidler, M. D., Nash, T. A., Kalt, W., Vinqvist-Tymchuk, M. R., Shukitt-Hale, B., & Joseph, J. A. (2010). Blueberry Supplementation Improves Memory in Older Adults. *Journal of Agricultural and Food Chemistry*, 58(7), 3996–4000. https://doi.org/10.1021/jf9029332

Ghasemzadeh Rahbardar, M., & Hosseinzadeh, H. (2020, September). *Therapeutic effects of rosemary (rosmarinus officinalis L.) and its active constituents on nervous system disorders*. Iranian journal of basic medical sciences. Retrieved February 7, 2022, from https://www.ncbi.nlm.nih.gov/pmc/articles/PMC7491497/

Ahmadpanah, M., Ramezanshams, F., Ghaleiha, A., Akhondzadeh, S., Sadeghi Bahmani, D., & Brand, S. (2019b). Crocus Sativus L. (saffron) versus sertraline on symptoms of depression among older people with major depressive disorders–a double-blind, randomized intervention study. *Psychiatry Research*, 282, 112613. https://doi.org/10.1016/j.psychres.2019.112613

Lipovac, M., Chedraui, P., Gruenhut, C., Gocan, A., Stammler, M., & Imhof, M. (2010). Improvement of postmenopausal depressive and anxiety symptoms after treatment with isoflavones derived from red clover extracts. *Maturitas*, 65(3), 258–261. https://doi.org/10.1016/j.maturitas.2009.10.014

Mansour, M. S., Ni, Y. M., Roberts, A. L., Kelleman, M., RoyChoudhury, A., & St-Onge, M. P. (2012). Ginger consumption enhances the thermic effect of food and promotes feelings of satiety without affecting metabolic and hormonal parameters in overweight men: A pilot study. *Metabolism*, 61(10), 1347–1352. https://doi.org/10.1016/j.metabol.2012.03.016

Ghanim, H., Sia, C. L., Abuaysheh, S., Korzeniewski, K., Patnaik, P., Marumganti, A., Chaudhuri, A., & Dandona, P. (2010). An Antiinflammatory and Reactive Oxygen Species Suppressive Effects of an Extract of Polygonum Cuspidatum Containing Resveratrol. *The Journal of Clinical Endocrinology & Metabolism*, 95(9), E1–E8. https://doi.org/10.1210/jc.2010-0482

Steiner, M., Khan, A. H., Holbert, D., & Lin, R. I. (1996). A double-blind crossover study in moderately hypercholesterolemic men that compared the effect of aged garlic extract and placebo administration on blood lipids. *The American Journal of Clinical Nutrition*, 64(6), 866–870. https://doi.org/10.1093/ajcn/64.6.866

Itchy skin (pruritus) - Symptoms and causes. (2021, January 6). Mayo Clinic. Retrieved January 13, 2022, from https://www.mayoclinic.org/diseases-conditions/itchy-skin/symptoms-causes/syc-20355006

Caflisch, K. M., Schmidt-Malan, S. M., Mandrekar, J. N., Karau, M. J., Nicklas, J. P., Williams, L. B., & Patel, R. (2018). Antibacterial activity of reduced iron clay against pathogenic bacteria associated with wound infections. *International Journal of Antimicrobial Agents*, 52(5), 692–696. https://doi.org/10.1016/j.ijantimicag.2018.07.018

Grimison, P., Mersiades, A., Kirby, A., Lintzeris, N., Morton, R., Haber, P., Olver, I., Walsh, A., McGregor, I., Cheung, Y., Tognela, A., Hahn, C., Briscoe, K., Aghmesheh, M., Fox, P., Abdi, E., Clarke, S., Della-Fiorentina, S., Shannon, J., . . . Stockler, M. (2020). Oral THC:CBD cannabis extract for refractory chemotherapy-induced nausea and vomiting: a randomised, placebo-controlled, phase II crossover trial. *Annals of Oncology*, 31(11), 1553–1560. https://doi.org/10.1016/j.annonc.2020.07.020

American Thyroid Association. (n.d.). Amiodarone. Retrieved from https://www.thyroid.org/amiodarone/

American Thyroid Association. (n.d.). Interferon alpha. Retrieved from https://www.thyroid.org/interferon-alpha/

American Thyroid Association. (n.d.). Tyrosine kinase inhibitors. Retrieved from https://www.thyroid.org/tyrosine-kinase-inhibitors/

Anti-seizure medications: American Thyroid Association. (n.d.). Anticonvulsant medications. Retrieved from https://www.thyroid.org/anticonvulsant-medications/

The Journal of Ethnopharmacology

The Journal of Allergy and Clinical Immunology

First time proof of sage's tolerability and efficacy in menopausal women with hot flushes (2016). Available at: https://www.ncbi.nlm.nih.gov/pmc/articles/PMC5044790/.

Chong, N. J., & Aziz, Z. (2012). A systematic review of the efficacy of Centella asiatica for improvement of the signs and symptoms of chronic venous insufficiency. Evidence-based complementary and alternative medicine : eCAM, 2013, 627182.

Shukla, A., Rasik, A. M., Jain, G. K., Shankar, R., & Kulshrestha, D. K. (1999). In vitro and in vivo wound healing activity of asiaticoside isolated from Centella asiatica. Journal of ethnopharmacology, 65(1), 1-11.

Rossi, A., Mari, E., Scarno, M., Gatti, A., & Lazzarini, R. (2009). Effects of saw palmetto extract on hair growth in men with androgenetic alopecia. Journal of Alternative and Complementary Medicine, 15(7), 1075-1079.

Belcaro, G., Cesarone, M. R., Dugall, M., Pellegrini, L., Ledda, A., Grossi, M. G., ... & Appendino, G. (2010). Product-evaluation registry of Meriva®, a curcumin-phosphatidylcholine complex, for the complementary management of osteoarthritis.

Panminerva medica, 52(2 Suppl 1), 55-62.

Cappello, G., Spezzaferro, M., Grossi, L., & Manzoli, L. (2007). Peppermint oil (Mintoil®) in the treatment of irritable bowel syndrome: a prospective double blind placebo-controlled randomized trial. Digestive and Liver Disease, 39(6), 530-536.

Wesnes, K. A., Ward, T., McGinty, A., & Petrini, O. (2000). The memory enhancing effects of a Ginkgo biloba/Panax ginseng combination in healthy middle-aged volunteers. Psychopharmacology, 152(4), 353-361.

Khan, A., Safdar, M., Ali Khan, M. M., Khattak, K. N., & Anderson, R. A. (2003). Cinnamon improves glucose and lipids of people with type 2 diabetes. Diabetes Care, 26(12), 3215-3218. doi: 10.2337/diacare.26.12.3215

Ranasinghe, P., Jayawardena, R., Galappaththy, P., Malkanthi, R., Constantine, G. R., & Katulanda, P. (2012). Efficacy and safety of 'true' cinnamon (Cinnamomum zeylanicum) as a pharmaceutical agent in diabetes: A systematic review and meta-analysis. Diabetic Medicine, 30(4), 505-512. doi: 10.1111/j.1464-5491.2012.03683.x

Neelakantan, N., Narayanan, M., de Souza, R. J., van Dam, R. M., & Mohan, V. (2014). Effect of fenugreek (Trigonella foenum-graecum L.) intake on glycemia: A meta-analysis of clinical trials. Nutrition Journal, 13(1), 7. doi: 10.1186/1475-2891-13-7

Madar, Z., & Abel, R. (1988). Glycemic response to fenugreek after different carbohydrate challenges in diabetics as compared to normal subjects. Israel Journal of Medical Sciences, 24(8), 437-441.

Baskaran, K., Ahamath, B. K., Shanmugasundaram, K. R., & Shanmugasundaram, E. R. (1990). Antidiabetic effect of a leaf extract from Gymnema sylvestre in non-insulin-dependent diabetes mellitus patients. Journal of Ethnopharmacology, 30(3), 295-300. doi: 10.1016/0378-8741(90)90101-2

Persaud, S. J., Al-Majed, H., Raman, A., & Jones, P. M. (1999). Gymnema sylvestre stimulates insulin release in vitro by increased membrane permeability. Journal of Endocrinology, 163(2), 207-212. doi: 10.1677/joe.0.1630207

Dans, A. M., Villarruz, M. V., Jimeno, C. A., Javelosa, M. A., Chua, J., Bautista, R., & Velez, G. G. (2007). The effect of Momordica charantia capsule preparation on glycemic control in type 2 diabetes mellitus needs further studies. Journal of Clinical Epidemiology, 60(6), 554-559. doi: 10.1016/j.jclinepi.2006.07.009

Ahmed, I., Adeghate, E., Cummings, E., & Sharma, A. K. (1998). Beneficial effects and mechanism of action of Momordica charantia juice in the treatment of streptozotocin-induced diabetes mellitus in rat. Molecular and Cellular Biochemistry, 181(1-2), 119-125.

Gupta, A. K., & Skinner, A. R. (2014). Management of recurrent vulvovaginal candidiasis: a review. Journal of Women's Health, 23(11), 895-902.

"What Causes Asthma?" - American Lung Association: https://www.lung.org/lung-health-diseases/lung-disease-lookup/asthma/learn-about-asthma/what-causes-asthma

"Asthma Causes and Triggers" - Mayo Clinic: https://www.mayoclinic.org/diseases-conditions/asthma/in-depth/asthma-triggers/art-20044382

"Non-allergic Asthma" - American Academy of Allergy, Asthma & Immunology: https://

www.aaaai.org/conditions-and-treatments/library/asthma-library/non-allergic-asthma

Ley, R. E., Peterson, D. A., & Gordon, J. I. (2006). Ecological and evolutionary forces shaping microbial diversity in the human intestine. Cell, 124(4), 837-848. doi: 10.1016/j.cell.2006.02.017

Round, J. L., & Mazmanian, S. K. (2009). The gut microbiota shapes intestinal immune responses during health and disease. Nature Reviews Immunology, 9(5), 313-323. doi: 10.1038/nri2515

Jandhyala, S. M., Talukdar, R., Subramanyam, C., Vuyyuru, H., Sasikala, M., & Reddy, D. N. (2015). Role of the normal gut microbiota. World Journal of Gastroenterology, 21(29), 8787-8803. doi: 10.3748/wjg.v21.i29.8787

U.S. National Library of Medicine. (2021, January 26). Probiotics. Retrieved from https://medlineplus.gov/probiotics.html

Li, Y., Poroyko, V., Yan, Z., Pan, L., Feng, Y., Zhao, P., . . . Wang, F. (2016). Characterization of intestinal microbiome in alcoholic patients with and without alcoholic hepatitis or cirrhosis. Scientific Reports, 6, 32341. doi: 10.1038/srep32341

Hu, F. B. (2011). Globalization of diabetes: The role of diet, lifestyle, and genes. Diabetes Care, 34(6), 1249-1257. doi: 10.2337/dc11-0442

Tillisch, K., Labus, J., Kilpatrick, L., Jiang, Z., Stains, J., Ebrat, B., . . . Mayer, E. A. (2013). Consumption of fermented milk product with probiotic modulates brain activity. Gastroenterology, 144(7), 1394-1401. doi: 10.1053/j.gastro.2013.02.043

National Institute of Diabetes and Digestive and Kidney Diseases. (2021, February). Digestive Diseases Statistics for the United States. Retrieved from https://www.niddk.nih.gov/health-information/health-statistics/digestive-diseases

National Center for Complementary and Integrative Health

Printed in Great Britain
by Amazon